Praise for Traditional Chinese
Medicine Approaches to Cancer
by Henry McGrath

'Chinese medicine has several important tools to offer in cancer management, but the cultural language and unique medical diagnosis can be a barrier to understanding the correct use of these tools. Henry McGrath has an excellent grasp on the true principles of Chinese medicine and he has managed to present it in a way that can be readily understood by cancer sufferers or specialists who seek to view this disease from another perspective.'

— Anthony Harrison,
former President of the Register of Chinese Herbal Medicine
and Director of the Register of Chinese Herbal Medicine
Chinese Herb Garden

'Henry McGrath has made great contributions to the improvement of professional education in Chinese medicine. In this much-needed book he clearly explains Chinese medicine to a lay audience. It shows that there is a solid research base behind the practice of Chinese medicine, and gives clear information to those with cancer.'

— Jeremy Ross,
Founder of Combining Western Herbs and Chinese Medicine Project
(Europe and North America)

'Henry McGrath has given us an invaluable gift. Taking the ancient and complex world of Chinese Medicine, he leads readers into a magical place of "Qi", of free flowing energy, harmony, balance and "whole person" therapy, in a ground-breaking and comprehensive study of this ancient medical system.

Here is information for the practitioner; hope for the cancer sufferer; and for the discerning reader a glimpse into the Tao: the path of spirituality; a way to wholeness, harmony and healing. This book will be of long term value to all who read it.'

— Pat Pilkington MBE,
Co-Founder, Penny Brohn Cancer Care

TRADITIONAL
CHINESE MEDICINE
APPROACHES *to* CANCER

of related interest

You Are How You Move
Experiential Chi Kung
Ged Sumner
ISBN 978 1 84819 014 6

Managing Depression with Qigong
Frances Gaik
ISBN 978 1 84819 018 4

Eternal Spring
Taijiquan, Qi Gong, and the Cultivation of Health, Happiness and Longevity
Michael W. Acton
ISBN 978 1 84819 003 0

HENRY McGRATH

TRADITIONAL
CHINESE MEDICINE
APPROACHES *to* CANCER

Harmony in the Face of the Tiger

SINGING DRAGON
London and Philadelphia

First published in 2009
by Singing Dragon
An imprint of Jessica Kingsley Publishers
116 Pentonville Road
London N1 9JB, UK
and
400 Market Street, Suite 400
Philadelphia, PA 19106, USA

www.singing-dragon.com

Library of Congress Cataloging in Publication Data
A CIP catalog record for this book is available from the Library of Congress

British Library Cataloguing in Publication Data
A CIP catalogue record for this book is available from the British Library

ISBN 978 1 84819 013 9

Printed and bound in the United States by
Thomson-Shore, 7300 Joy Road, Dexter, MI 48130

CONTENTS

ACKNOWLEDGMENTS

Words cannot express how much this book owes to my wife Mariola, for her editing skills, for taking more than her share of domestic responsibilities so that I could write, and most importantly for teaching me so much about love.

Thanks to my children, Carl, Miriam and Thea, for endless joy and inspiration.

Thanks to my parents, for a lifetime of love and support.

Thanks to Philip Ashton, for input on research.

Thanks to Phil Cooper for help with the illustrations.

Thanks to Zhang Zhi Chen in Beijing, for looking after me in China, and for help with research and translation.

Thanks to Professor Ursula King, who was so helpful in getting this book published.

Thanks to all the staff at Penny Brohn Cancer Care.

Thanks to all the staff and students at the College of Naturopathic Medicine.

Thanks to all my patients, who have taught me so much.

HOW TO USE THIS BOOK

CHAPTER 1: **The Chinese Understanding of Cancer** • This chapter gives an introduction to Chinese medicine and its understanding of cancer, allowing you to understand the rest of the book. It can be used again for reference as you read the other chapters, especially if you need to clarify the underlying theories.

CHAPTER 2: **Cultivating the Spirit: The Psychology of Chinese Medicine** • This chapter is an introduction to the philosophies underpinning Chinese medicine, particularly as they relate to cancer. It can be used to enhance personal growth and development, and to help one reflect on the "cancer journey". References are given for those who wish to explore further.

CHAPTER 3: **Celestial Lancets: Acupuncture in the Management of Cancer** • This chapter gives insight into what acupuncture can do for those with cancer, backing this up with some of the latest research. It discusses the theoretical basis for acupuncture, and also how it works from a scientific perspective. It gives information about finding an acupuncturist, and will help you gain a deeper understanding of your acupuncture treatment.

CHAPTER 4: **Elixir of Life: Herbal Medicine in the Management of Cancer** • This chapter shows how herbal medicine is integrated into cancer treatment in China, and gives insight into what herbal medicine can do for those with cancer. It presents some of the latest research into the anti-cancer properties of some Chinese herbs. It gives information about finding a Chinese herbalist, and will help you to gain a deeper understanding of your herbal treatment.

Chapter 5: **Nourishing the Soul: The Chinese Approach to Nutrition** • This chapter can best be used once you have a Traditional Chinese Medicine diagnosis, which you should obtain from your acupuncturist and/or Chinese herbalist. You can then use this diagnosis to select the appropriate kinds of foods discussed in this chapter. This chapter explains that the Chinese approach is to select foods which are appropriate to your own, individual diagnosis.

Chapter 6: **Cultivating Qi** • This chapter discusses the benefits of exercises called "Qi Gong", which are designed to strengthen your energy and calm your mind. It will help you to select a qualified practitioner who can help you do the exercises.

This chapter shows how problems in our relationship to the environment and the wider cosmos can contribute to cancer. It introduces the Chinese art of "Feng Shui", which is a system for harmonising one's relationship to the environment. It helps you find a practitioner of Feng Shui.

Please note that this book is in no way a substitute for consulting properly qualified and experienced practitioners.

An Integrated Approach

Western medicine has made great strides in treating many kinds of cancer. Powerful new drugs have been developed that kill cancer cells. Surgical techniques have been refined, making it possible to cut out many kinds of cancer. As a result, a huge number of people are surviving cancer.[1]

While western medicine has had many successes in dealing with cancer itself, it does not focus on the person. By concentrating solely on the disease, it tends to miss the human being involved. It does not attempt to sustain people through the harrowing process of diagnosis, treatment and recovery. It does not equip people to face the challenging issues that a cancer diagnosis brings. There is a need for something more in our approach to cancer.

The Chinese approach is the perfect complement to orthodox treatment. It focuses on the whole person, and seeks to sustain her on the journey through cancer and beyond. It attempts to strengthen the body and to nurture the spirit, giving renewed vitality and hope. The following comments give a flavour of how some of my patients have experienced Chinese medicine:

> You are the first person who has actually *looked* at me. I mean, *all* of me.

---

1   *Macmillan Cancer Survivors' Guide*, 2009.

It's such a relief to be able to tell someone my whole story.

I always knew that losing my mother was the start of my cancer. Doctors never wanted to hear that, but *you* can see how it fits into the story. It's good to know I'm not just imagining it.

Chinese medicine makes all the parts of my cancer join up. It helps me make sense of it.

With Chinese medicine I feel like I can do something for myself at last. I can start to help myself, instead of just being told 'take this, take that'.

One of the reasons why western medicine has saved the lives of so many people with cancer is that the oncologist has specialised. Each consultant has an incredible depth of knowledge in his particular field. Hospitals are divided into specialist departments, allowing great progress to be made in each area. Specialist laboratory techniques have analysed and classified the various kinds of tumour tissue. However, the converse of this approach is that no doctor looks at the whole person, and gets the full picture. A consultant oncologist is not interested in patients' diets, their personal relationships, their emotional lives, their careers, or their homes. Indeed, he is barely interested in their physical body as a whole: he sees only a tumour.

Patients often tell me that they encounter a variety of health professionals, all of whom look at different parts of them. The consultant oncologist looks at their tumour. The endocrinologist measures their hormone levels. They are referred to a pain clinic for their pains, and advised to see a counsellor for their depression. They may be referred to a neurologist if their nerves are affected by chemotherapy, and an immunologist if their immune system is affected. Sometimes patients are given conflicting advice by the various specialists, and many struggle to integrate the various pieces of information which they are presented with.

Many patients feel as though they are falling between various nets, and that no one person is holding them.

This fragmented approach is reinforced by the nature of research in western medicine. Controlled trials are set up which measure the impact of a certain drug on one variable, which in the case of cancer is the size of the tumour in the short term. The impact of the drug on the whole person is deliberately excluded from such trials. No attempt is made to address the other factors which may have contributed to the cancer, such as liver malfunction, digestive problems, blood disorders, immune disorders, endocrine disorders or emotional factors. The very nature of western medicine is not to treat the person, but to treat the disease. Indeed, it does not even attempt to treat the whole disease, but treats only the most obvious and easily measurable aspect of the disease, which is the tumour itself.

Western medicine does not tend to focus on the causes of disease: it focuses instead on their manifestation. For example, although much research has been done into the role of diet in the formation of cancer, this does not form part of the orthodox approach. Very rarely have I heard of an oncologist offering dietary advice to cancer patients.

Although we successfully treat a larger proportion of certain cancers, by ignoring their causes the overall numbers of many cancers are rising at an astronomical rate. For example breast cancer incidence rates have increased by more than 50 per cent over the last 25 years.[2] This is a huge and worrying trend, and one wonders where it will end. At this rate of increase it will not be too long before a huge majority of women get breast cancer. And yet we are continuing to focus only on treating the cancer, rather than trying also to understand the causes of it. We are fighting the fire, but forgetting to put away the matches.

---

2   Cancer Research UK.

None of this is to argue that traditional Chinese medicine is an alternative to western medicine. It is, however, to say that Chinese medicine is its perfect complement. Western medicine has a micro approach, focusing inwards on the fine detail of cancer cells: Chinese medicine has a macro approach, focusing on the whole person, and outwards to their environment. Western medicine focuses on the disease: Chinese medicine focuses on the person, looking in great detail at all aspects of his life, mental and physical. The practitioner of Chinese medicine takes a careful note of all bodily functions, such as sleep patterns, diet, digestion, and emotional factors. It examines the patient's tongue and pulse in great detail. It builds up a complete picture of a unique human being. It tries to understand why a disease has arisen, and therefore how it can be treated, and recurrence prevented. It seeks to understand the patient's story, and how her disease fits into that story. Illness is never seen in isolation, but as part of a pattern.

It has sometimes been said that western medicine sees the human person as a soulless machine. This view has a tendency to become self-fulfilling: if we are treated like machines for long enough, we start to feel like machines. If one forgets the soul, sure enough the soul will shrink. Chinese medicine, on the other hand, retains a vision of each human person as a unique integration of body and mind. This means that we can only understand disease as part of the full human picture, not in isolation.

Chinese medicine sees the human person in relation to her surroundings. We can only be fully understood as part of a social network, and as part of mankind. By focusing on the human purely as an individual, we diminish what it means to be human. This has become another self-fulfilling prophecy: we are becoming a collection of autonomous individuals, rather than an integrated society. This is seen all too clearly in many people with cancer, who are left feeling very isolated. Chinese medicine reminds us that our relationships with others are a key part of our health.

In this book we shall see that Chinese medicine provides many cost effective and sustainable ways to manage the side effects of western cancer treatments. When orthodox treatment is over, it can help people to regain strength and vitality, and to take back control over their lives. When people complete their cancer treatment, many are left thinking:

> I have survived this far: what next? Do I just sit around waiting for the next set of tests? How do I rebuild my life? What can I do to try and ensure the cancer does not come back?

This book shows how Chinese medicine addresses these questions, and helps people through the long and painful process of cancer and beyond, living their lives as fully as possible, for as long as possible.

In some parts of our health services the Chinese approach is already being well integrated: this process should be accelerated, for the benefit of all people with cancer.

CHAPTER ONE

The Chinese Understanding of Cancer

CHAPTER CONTENTS

Introduction • Qi: the life force • Eight Principles diagnosis • The Chinese organ system • The Five Elements • The causes of disease • Tongue diagnosis • Pulse diagnosis • Summary

INTRODUCTION

The theoretical basis of Chinese medicine goes back to a few centuries BC, and much of it is outlined in a book called *The Yellow Emperor's Classic of Medicine*, written at that time.[3] The book takes the form of the Yellow Emperor asking questions of his Minister, Qi Bo, about health matters. The Yellow Emperor asks why people only live to be fifty years old nowadays, whereas those who lived in the past lived to be around one hundred. Qi Bo replies that:

> In the past, people practised the Tao, the Way of Life. They understood the principle of balance, of yin and yang, as represented by the transformation of the energies of the universe.

---

3   Ni, M (1995) *The Yellow Emperor's Classic of Medicine*. Boston, MA: Shambhala.

Thus, they formulated practices such as Dao-In, an exercise combining stretching, massaging, and breathing to promote energy flow, and meditation to help maintain and harmonise themselves with the universe. They ate a balanced diet at regular times, arose and retired at regular hours, avoided over stressing their bodies and minds, and refrained from over indulgence of all kinds. They maintained well-being of body and mind; thus it is not surprising that they lived over one hundred years.

Qi Bo goes on to outline how people have changed their way of life:

They drink wine as though it were water, indulge excessively in destructive activities, drain their jing – the body's essence that is stored in the kidneys – and deplete their qi. They do not know the secret of conserving their energy and vitality. Seeking emotional excitement and momentary pleasures, people disregard the natural rhythm and order of the universe. They fail to regulate their lifestyle and diet, and sleep improperly. So it is not surprising that they look old at fifty and die soon thereafter.

This passage summarises the approach of Chinese medicine. The practitioner of Chinese medicine will try to guide the patient back to a way of living which is more in keeping with the Natural Order. Although Chinese medicine uses techniques, such as herbs and acupuncture, to help the patient, the key to returning to full health is to change one's way of living. Chinese medicine is not just a set of techniques; it is a way of life and a philosophy. This philosophy consists of living in harmony with those around us, and with the planet. Chinese medicine has a strong ecological basis, which resonates particularly with our times. It assumes that the universe, part of which is our planet, is arranged in a harmonious way, and that we are called to live in tune with that harmony. We shall look in more detail at the philosophy of Chinese medicine in the chapter on cultivating the spirit, and we shall see that this philosophy is not inconsistent with any religion.

The analysis of Qi Bo has much to tell us all. If he was shocked at the dissolute and stressful lifestyle of ancient China, how much more shocked would he be at our lifestyles?

Qi Bo recognised that a disease such as cancer was very serious. He did not offer miracle cures, and outlined many situations where Chinese medicine could do little to save the patient. We now have stronger medical techniques than existed in ancient China, and although this is good in itself, the fact that so many of us need these powerful interventions reflects how sick we have become. In Qi Bo's day, acupuncture and herbs were regarded as strong medical interventions, and the need to use them reflected a very serious imbalance. How much more so with chemotherapy, radiotherapy and surgery?

We shall see in this book that, far from holding an outmoded view of the human person, Chinese medicine offers profound insights into what makes us well, in the fullest sense of the word. Rather than seeing the human being as an isolated unit, it shows us how we are intimately enmeshed in our environment, and that our health depends crucially on our surroundings. The human person is a reflection of the whole universe, a microcosm of the entire cosmos. What happens "out there" influences what happens "in here".

The reverse is equally true: human actions have a profound influence on the rest of the planet, and even of the whole cosmos. When humanity falls, the rest of creation falls with us.[4]

According to the Chinese view, the human person is not just a collection of parts, put together like a machine. The human person is a fully integrated being, with all parts intimately connected to each other. The physical body is inseparable from the

---

4   This insight was recognised by the Church Fathers of the Christian tradition too.

mind, and *the whole is far more than the sum of the parts.* We shall see in this book that problems in the mind are reflected in physical problems, and vice versa. Chinese medicine therefore seeks to build up a picture of the whole person, rather than just focusing on the part that appears to be "broken".

We shall also find that the Chinese understanding is increasingly backed by modern research, which has confirmed much of what the ancient Chinese had worked out by other means. We are now coming to realise in the West that a disease such as cancer is a complex entity, caused by several factors occurring together. These factors can include emotions, diet, internal biological factors, and the environment. However, this appreciation that cancer is a complex disease, reflecting imbalances in the whole human organism, has not yet been reflected in our approach to cancer, which still sees a tumour as an isolated entity which can be cut out or poisoned. In this book we shall see how the Chinese understanding of the human being allows us to treat the whole person. Chinese medicine seeks to address all of the factors involved in cancer, as these manifest in each unique human being.

In order to see how Chinese medicine can help us gain a deeper understanding of cancer, we must first explore in some detail the Chinese understanding of the human person. This chapter will outline some of the basic theories of Chinese medicine, which will allow us to see, in the rest of the book, what it can offer those with cancer.

QI: THE LIFE FORCE

The concept of "qi" is fundamental to an understanding of Chinese medicine. There is no direct translation of this word, but the closest we can come is perhaps the idea of a life force. Qi is the animating principle of life. The amount and quality of qi determines how healthy and full of vitality one is. If a person is full of energy, in robust health, and with a positive outlook, we say they have strong qi. If a person is always tired, feels weak, is often ill, we say they have weak qi. In this book, we will explore many ways to cultivate strong qi, which is vital in the fight against cancer.

The human person is intimately connected to the outside world through constant exchange of qi. We take in fresh qi when we breathe in, and expel stale qi when we breathe out. Food contains qi, and we must try to take in food with good quality qi. This means food which is fresh, and not full of chemicals. When food is refined and processed the qi is destroyed.

The quality of our personal relationships has a profound impact on our qi, as we are constantly exchanging qi with those around us. If we are surrounded by a loving family, our qi is strengthened. If, on the other hand, somebody is angry with us, or makes us feel tired, they are draining our qi. If we are surrounded by an atmosphere of stress, at home or at work, our qi will suffer.

We absorb qi from the place where we live. If we live in a calm, nourishing, clean place, our qi is supported. If we live in a noisy, dirty, polluted place, our qi is drained.

Qi is neither fully *matter*, nor fully *energy*. Put another way, it is neither purely *material*, nor purely *non-material*. It is neither body, nor mind, but something in between. Qi acts as a kind of interface between the material world, and the non-material world, between the body and the mind. In the human person, the mind influences the qi, and in turn the qi influences the body. Likewise, the body influences the qi, and the qi influences the mind.

The concept of qi gives a new dimension to the ecological issue. If we destroy the qi of the planet, we destroy our own qi.

This is why Chinese medicine is ecological medicine: we must keep the planet healthy in order for us to remain healthy.

Qi flows through the body in channels, which we call "meridians". The meridians start at the tips of the fingers and toes, and then flow into the organs. In addition, the meridians all flow into each other in one large circuit. If the qi flows freely, the organs will be healthy. If the qi flow is blocked, the organs will become ill.

There are 12 main meridians, each linked to an organ. We shall learn more about these meridians in the chapter on acupuncture. The job of the acupuncturist is to encourage the healthy flow of qi.

One can talk about qi in a *general* sense, and say that qi flows throughout the universe. There are also *specific* kinds of qi, for example human qi is different to plant qi. With Chinese medicine we need to study the properties of *human* qi, which we shall now do.

The properties of human qi

1. QI WARMS

One of the characteristics of humans is our warmth, which distinguishes us from cold blooded animals and plants. If we have good qi, we feel comfortably warm. If we have weak qi, we will feel too cold. As we shall see later, cold can give rise to health problems, and can be a contributory factor in the development of certain cancers.

2. QI MOVES

Another characteristic of humans is movement: qi allows us to move. If we have lots of qi, we will have plenty of energy to move around. If we lack qi, we will be slow and sluggish. Qi is also the force which moves substances around inside our bodies. If we have strong qi, we can move our food properly though the digestive tract, and distribute our blood and fluids properly. If we have weak qi, our digestion will be sluggish, our blood circulation may be poor, and we may get problems with our fluid metabolism. On a cellular level, our cells may not get the nutrients they need, and may not be able to excrete wastes properly. Toxins may build up, which can be one of the factors contributing to cancer.

3. QI PROTECTS

Qi protects us from illness: if we have strong qi, we tend to get ill rarely, and our illnesses tend to be mild. Qi is the force which attacks any pathogens in the body, and prevents them from developing. Strong qi is therefore vital in the fight against cancer.

4. QI TRANSFORMS

Qi allows the transformation of food into more qi, in a kind of virtuous circle. If we have strong qi, we can make more qi. Qi also allows the transformation of food into blood. The Chinese conception of blood is somewhat different from the modern orthodox perspective, and is outlined below in the section on "blood deficiency". From a western perspective, we can say that qi breaks food down into nutrients, and promotes the absorption of those nutrients into the blood, for distribution to the cells. If our qi is strong, we will be able to digest our food well, and absorb and assimilate the nutrients. If our qi is weak, we will not absorb all the nutrients from our food. Even if we have a good diet, our body will lack key nutrients. So what happens to the undigested food? According to Chinese medicine, it is stored around the body as a substance we call "phlegm". Phlegm is a pathogenic substance, which can form tumours if other factors are present (we will look at phlegm in more detail below). For this reason, strong qi is vital in preventing and managing cancer.

5. QI HOLDS AND RAISES

Qi is the force which allows us to be upright. It is the force which allows everything in the body to be held in place. If the qi is weak, we may suffer from prolapse, or we may feel heavy or sluggish. On a mental level, we may feel unsupported, or even a sense of collapse. We may be unable to *raise* our spirits. Restoring the qi is therefore vital in helping to restore a sense of hope and optimism in those with cancer.

Qi pathologies

There are two qi pathologies. Firstly, there is *qi deficiency*, where there is simply not enough qi in the body. Secondly, there is *qi stagnation*. With this pathology, the person may have enough qi, but the qi flow is blocked. Causes of qi stagnation include emotional problems and stress. When the qi stagnates, all the functions of qi are impeded.

Unfortunately, chemotherapy and radiotherapy often deplete the qi, so it is essential that patients receiving these treatments find ways to maintain their qi.

In summary, we can see that one of the key elements in the fight against cancer is the cultivation of qi. We will see throughout the book that there are many ways to do this.

EIGHT PRINCIPLES DIAGNOSIS

In order for effective treatment and advice to be given, a correct diagnosis must be made. One of the strengths of Chinese medicine is its advanced diagnostic tools. I am often asked to recommend particular herbs, foods, or advice for people with cancer. However, this is impossible without having first done a diagnosis. As mentioned above, Chinese medicine recognises many different patterns of cancer, and it is essential to identify which pattern is present in any individual before treatment can begin.

One of the main ways in which we make a diagnosis is according to a model known as the "Eight Principles". This model classifies illness according to four pairs of opposites, as follows:

yang	**yin**
heat	**cold**
excess	**deficiency**
external	**internal**

The principles on the left are the four yang principles, and the principles on the right are the four yin principles. Before we can go further we need to explain the concept of yang and yin.

Yang and yin

According to Chinese medicine, the whole universe is composed of two opposite principles, yang and yin. These principles interact to give the universe shape, dynamism, and the capacity to change. According to Chinese cosmology, before the moment of creation, everything was undifferentiated. Creation occurred when the One became two, which allowed structure, change and movement. We had day and night, male and female, energy and matter. These two opposites, yang and yin, work together harmoniously, interplaying with each other, supporting each other, but never merging. It is like a husband and wife: in one sense they are united, by helping and caring for each other. But in another sense, they remain separate. When yang and yin are harmonious, it is like a good marriage, with mutual support, communication and understanding. When yang and yin are out of harmony, it is like a bad marriage, where communication breaks down, and each person struggles on in isolation.

Yang and yin are rooted in the very structure of the universe: an atom is composed of a yin part and a yang part. The nucleus has the yin properties of being still, material, heavy, and internal. The electron whizzing around the nucleus has the opposite yang properties of movement, energy, lightness and externality.

As it is in the cosmos (the macrocosm), so it is in the human person (the microcosm). When yang and yin are in harmony, we are healthy. When they are out of harmony, we are ill. *All illness can be understood as a disharmony of yang and yin.*

The next stage is to look at yang and yin in more detail, as it works in the human person. This is where we come back to the Eight Principles, which we listed above. The fundamental qualities of yang in the human person are hot, excess, and external. The qualities of yin are cold, deficiency, and internal. So, for example, one kind of illness may consist of too much heat in one part of the body, and too much cold in another part. If yang and yin were in harmony, this would not occur, because the heat and cold would interact. The heat would go where it was needed, and the cold would go where it was needed. But when the husband and wife are not communicating, the heat stays locked in one room, and the cold stays locked in another. For example, a person could have heat in the liver, but cold in the uterus. Or, to give another example, a person could have an *excess* of fluids in the lower body (oedema), and a *deficiency* of fluids in the upper body (a dry cough).

The task of the practitioner is to determine exactly in what way yang and yin are out of balance in a particular person, and then to restore that balance. One must identify which parts are too hot, and which parts are too cold. One must determine which parts are in excess, and which deficient. Is the disease external, or internal?

We can see that this is a fundamentally *holistic* model of health, as we need to examine the situation in the whole body, not just the diseased part. In a sense, no illness is ever confined to one area: when yang and yin are out of balance, the *whole person* is always affected, and the whole person must always be treated. A tumour is never seen in isolation from the rest of the person, as something that can merely be cut out. It is but the physical manifestation of an imbalance of the whole person.

The whole person includes the mind (which is yang), and body (which is yin). If one aspect is out of balance, the other will be affected. All disease is, to a greater or lesser extent, both physical and mental. This is why Chinese medicine always seeks to work on both body and mind. Illness may start in the body, but will end up affecting the mind too. Or illness may start in the mind, but will end up affecting the body too.

If we think of cancer, it may be caused by primarily physical factors which affect the body, such as pollution, genetics, or diet. However, eventually the mind will be affected: the person will experience anger, anxiety, grief, or other emotions. Conversely, the person may start with an emotional/psychological problem, which affects the physical body. As we said, a problem with yang will always become a problem with yin too, and vice versa. A husband who is an alcoholic will bring trouble for the wife. A wife who is depressed will bring trouble for the husband. Being a practitioner of Chinese medicine is a little like being a marriage guidance counsellor: always trying to help the parties towards mutual co-operation and understanding, and trying to prevent a divorce. The further yang and yin are separated from each other, the worse the illness becomes. Total separation of yang and yin is the end of the road: divorce and death.

So how do we establish which particular pattern of disharmony is present in any individual? How do we know which parts are hot, which parts are cold, which parts are excess, and which are deficient? We have looked at yang and yin, the two governing principles which contain the other principles. Let us now look in more detail at the three yang principles, and the three yin principles. As we mentioned, these principles are pairs of opposites.

Heat (yang) and cold (yin)

HEAT

Heat causes expansion, so hot diseases are often associated with swelling, such as prostate hypertrophy, or rheumatoid arthritis. We can also think of inflammatory conditions as hot diseases. These often end in "itis", such as hepatitis, cystitis, or meningitis. With these kinds of diseases, the patient often feels overheated, or feels a burning sensation in the affected area.

Heat causes things to go too fast, and so hot diseases often involve hyper-function, which is where some part of the body is working too fast. For example, hyperthyroidism is when the thyroid is working too hard, causing the metabolism to go too fast. With this condition, people burn up calories very quickly, and can be underweight. They will often have an excess of nervous energy, and suffer anxiety or insomnia.

Heat dries up the body fluids, so patients with hot conditions often have concentrated fluids, such as dark urine. The lack of fluids may cause the stools to be dry, possibly leading to constipation. The concentration of fluids may cause the urine and stools to smell strongly.

Heat is said to agitate the mind, so these patients may suffer from agitation, restlessness, or insomnia. They may display hot emotions, such as anger or irritability.

Often the person will say that they feel overheated, and need to open all the windows. These people will often be found outside in winter with very few clothes on.

People who are predominantly hot will tend to be red in colour, especially in the face. They will tend to have red tongues. Their pulses will often be rapid, signifying a rapid metabolism.

The table on p.31 gives a summary of the signs of hot pathologies.

So what are the *causes* of heat? In Chinese medicine, food and drink are classified according to whether they have properties of heating and cooling. Hot pathologies can be caused by the consumption of too many heating substances, such as alcohol, drugs (prescribed or illegal), certain spices, fried food, and certain food additives.

Strong emotions may also cause heat, particularly anger, frustration and stress. Our fast paced modern lives cause us to overheat: we are always on the move, and lack calmness and rest.

When heat is present for a long period of time, it can cause chronic inflammatory conditions, such as colitis (bowel inflammation), or ulceration. This situation results in a breakdown of proper movement of blood, fluids, and the inadequate clearing of waste products. In Chinese medicine we say that "stagnation" is occurring. From a western perspective, we would say that cells are not receiving the proper nutrients, and are not excreting waste products properly. In Chinese medicine we say that "*heat toxins*" are accumulating. This is potentially a dangerous situation, and is often one of the key factors in the development of cancer.

COLD

With cold conditions, patients often feel very cold, and find it hard to get warm. These people will want to wear lots of warm clothes, sit near the radiator, and drink lots of hot drinks.

Cold causes things to slow down, and move sluggishly. It causes matter to coagulate, which prevents it moving properly. We can use the analogy of a soup placed in the fridge, which becomes thick and lumpy, with fats coagulating on the surface.

Because cold slows things down, cold conditions often involve *hypo*-function (under-function), such as hypothyroidism. This is where the metabolism is too slow, and the person lacks energy. They find it difficult to burn calories, and can easily become overweight.

Cold people tend to have copious body fluids, because there is a lack of heat to dry the fluids. Their urine will tend to be pale and copious. Their stools may be loose and watery.

Emotionally, they will tend to be cooler, more introverted, perhaps prone to depression or grief. They will often lack vitality and energy. They may be apathetic and unmotivated.

Often these people will have a pale complexion and a pale tongue. The tongue may also be swollen, reflecting the excess amount of fluids. The pulse will often be slow in these people, reflecting a slow metabolism.

So what are the *causes* of cold? They include living in a cold climate; allowing oneself to become too cold; eating foods and drinks with cold properties, such as raw foods and chilled drinks. Cold may be caused by emotional factors, such as not receiving loving warmth.

Cold is one of the main factors involved in the development of many kinds of cancer. When the body is cold, there is a lack of movement and things tend to stagnate. Energy cannot flow freely around the body. Fluids accumulate, and can cause "phlegm" in the body. As we shall see later, the build up of phlegm can be an important factor in the development of certain cancers.

In many pathologies, some parts of the body may be too hot, while others are too cold. The heat remains stuck in one part, and the cold stuck in another part. We can also note that cold conditions can transform into hot ones, and vice versa. For example, cold may lead to stagnation, which may then lead to the build up of heat toxins.

Summary of the main signs of hot and cold pathologies

	Signs of hot pathologies	Signs of cold pathologies
Colour (including face)	Red	Pale
Subjective feeling	Hot	Cold
Climate preferred	Cold	Hot
Clothing	Wears less	Wears more
Thirst	Strong	Absent
Drinks preferred	Cold	Hot
Metabolism	Fast	Slow
Hunger	Strong	Weak
Sleep	Disturbed	Likes to curl up
Body secretions	Thick/scanty yellow/smelly	Thin/copious clear/no smell
Stools	Constipation	Loose
Pain better for	Cold	Warmth (e.g. hot water bottle)
Fluids	Dry	Damp
Tongue	Red body/red spots Maybe yellow coat	Pale/bluish/maybe swollen
Pulse	Rapid	Slow

Excess (yang) and deficiency (yin)

EXCESS

The Chinese concept of "excess" refers to a situation where too much of something is present. A cancer tumour by definition is an excess pattern: something is there which should not be there.

The disease pattern in our society is very different from that seen in the third world. In pre-industrial societies, much disease is caused by *deficiency*, in particular a lack of nutrients. By contrast, many western diseases are caused by an *excess* amount of certain things. It is interesting, and perhaps ironic, that as countries such as China industrialise, and become more "prosperous", many kinds of cancers are rapidly increasing.

The main factors which tend to be in excess are known as the "Four Fullnesses", and these are:

1. Damp.

2. Phlegm.

3. Food.

4. Stagnant blood.

We will look at each of these in turn.

The Four Fullnesses

1. PHLEGM. We have already mentioned phlegm above. The Chinese concept of phlegm is a much broader concept than ours. It refers to a fixed accumulation of material anywhere in the body. According to Chinese medicine, phlegm is primarily generated in the digestive system. It consists of food which the body has been unable to break down properly, and which is stored in the tissues. We can think of choles-

terol as a kind of phlegm. Phlegm also includes fat tissue, as well as all kinds of lumps. These lumps may be benign or malign. According to Chinese medicine, phlegm is one of the main causes of cancer. Phlegm is known as the "cause of a thousand diseases".

If someone's digestive system is weak, they will be prone to phlegm. Certain foods can lead to the formation of phlegm in some people, particularly dairy products, wheat and fried foods (we will look at this in more detail in the chapter on nutrition). From a western perspective, certain people lack the enzymes to digest these foods effectively. As one gets older, one produces less digestive enzymes, and so one becomes more prone to phlegm.

2. DAMP. As we mentioned above, people who are cold will often accumulate excessive fluids in their tissues. Chinese medicine refers to this condition as damp. From a western perspective, one can think of oedema. Often one of the side effects of cancer treatment is ascites, which is a build of up fluids. An excessive amount of damp in the body can lead to the formation of phlegm.

3. FOOD. In our society many people simply eat too much food. If one always has large meals, the body may be unable to digest all the food. This food will tend to sit in the digestive tract, and not get broken down properly. This can lead to the build up of phlegm.

4. STAGNANT BLOOD. This Chinese concept refers to a situation where the micro-circulation of the blood is impaired. This concept also corresponds to what western doctors call "sticky blood". With *blood stagnation*, nutrients from the blood do not get into the cells efficiently, and cellular waste products are not taken into the blood efficiently. Along with phlegm, blood stagnation is one of the main causes of cancer.

DEFICIENCY

We have said that tumours are, by definition, excess patterns. However, while the tumour itself may be an excess, the *causes* of the tumour usually involve some kind of deficiency. Western medicine is often effective in removing the tumour itself, but does not address the deficiency aspects which may have caused the tumour. For example, we have seen that a *deficiency* of qi can lead to a build up of *excess* phlegm. Or a *deficiency* of qi can lead to the *excess* pattern of blood stagnation, because there is not enough qi to move the blood properly. It is this focus on the whole person, on the whole pattern, which makes Chinese medicine truly holistic. The tumour itself is just the manifestation of a bigger picture.

It is therefore vital to establish the underlying deficiencies which may have contributed to the tumour. Chinese medicine recognises the "Four Deficiencies", which are:

1. Qi deficiency.

2. Blood deficiency.

3. Yang deficiency.

4. Yin deficiency.

Let us now look in more detail at each of these deficiencies.

The Four Deficiencies

1. QI DEFICIENCY. We have already looked at this pattern above, in the section on qi.

2. BLOOD DEFICIENCY. This is where there are inadequate nutrients in the blood. The blood is deficient not so much in terms of the *quantity* of blood, but more in terms of the *quality* of blood. Nutrient deficiency comes from two sources:

inadequate nutrients in the *diet*, and inadequate *absorption* of nutrients. The patient, under the guidance of the practitioner, must ensure they have the right diet, based on their diagnostic pattern (this is examined in more depth in the nutrition chapter). In addition, the qi of the patient must be cultivated in order to maximise the amount of nutrients that are absorbed. Remember, *it is the strength of one's qi that determines the amount of food absorbed.*

The Chinese concept of blood is broader than the orthodox western concept of blood, and a proper distinction should be made between blood as defined by Chinese medicine, and blood as defined by western medicine. According to the Chinese conception, blood has three functions:

1. **Blood nourishes:** As with orthodox western medicine, blood carries nutrients to every part of the body. Those patients who are "blood deficient" will tend to look pale, dry, and perhaps withered. Blood deficiency is a major contributory factor in some kinds of cancer: if inadequate nutrients reach the cells, they cannot function optimally, and so are more prone to becoming cancerous.

2. **Blood moistens:** If the blood is deficient, the patient will tend to be dry. This may manifest in dry skin, or in dry stools and constipation.

3. **Blood supports the emotions:** When the blood is rich in nutrients, the person will feel emotionally balanced. If the blood is deficient, the person may feel anxious or nervous, and find that their sleep is disturbed. Often a diagnosis of cancer will have a profound emotional impact, so it is necessary to nourish the blood to support the emotions.

Radiotherapy is said to dry the blood, and can sometimes lead to blood deficiency. It is therefore often necessary to nourish the blood, particularly if blood deficiency was one of the contributory factors to the cancer.

3. YANG DEFICIENCY. We have seen that yang is warming, energising, and stimulating. People with yang deficiency will therefore tend to be cold, tired, and apathetic. They will tend to be more introverted, and experience "cold" emotions, such as grief and fear. They may find it hard to get started, especially in the morning, and may need to drink lots of coffee to keep going. If the condition is extreme, they may develop chronic fatigue. Because there is a lack of internal movement, they may be prone to developing phlegm, blood stagnation, and toxic build up.

Case history of yang deficiency: Jean, aged 62

Jean was diagnosed with breast cancer. She underwent a mastectomy, and received chemotherapy and radiotherapy. She was also found to have large cysts in her uterus, but these were not cancerous. She suffered from severe weight gain, which she found very hard to shift. She had suffered from chronic fatigue and depression for many years, and this had led to her early retirement on medical grounds. She really hated the cold, which made her feel even more tired and depressed.

In terms of Chinese medicine, the background to her cancer was yang deficiency. The yang principle warms, and gives a sense of vitality. Because she lacked yang, she felt cold, tired, sluggish and depressed. There was not enough yang to move the fluids around properly, so she had accumulated a lot of damp and phlegm, which accounted for her weight gain, as well as the breast tumour and cysts.

After acupuncture, Jean felt more energy, and felt more positive mentally. After a course of treatment she had developed enough motivation and energy to begin exercising, and began to lose weight. She was also feeling warmer: part of her treatment had involved burning a herb (called Artemisia) near to acupuncture points, which has a warming effect.

4. YIN DEFICIENCY. We have seen that yin is cooling, relaxing, and calming. People with yin deficiency will therefore tend to be overheated, unable to relax and to "switch off". They may be workaholics, unable to stop. They may be unable to wind down in the evening, and find it hard to go to sleep. They will tend to experience "hot" emotions, such as irritability and anger.

As we have said, problems of yang will eventually cause problems with yin. With an advanced pathology such as cancer, most people are deficient in both yang and yin. These people will find it hard to get started, but hard to switch off. They will feel too cold sometimes, and too hot at other times. Too much yang will rise up, causing heat and dryness in the upper body. This is often an issue with cancers of the upper body, such as breast and stomach cancer. Correspondingly, too much yin will sink down, causing dampness, cold, and stagnation in the lower body. This can lead to the build up of phlegm. This is often the case with cancers in the lower body, such as colon, uterine, cervical and prostate.

Case history of yin deficiency: Jane, aged 55

Jane was diagnosed with cancer of the throat. She underwent an operation to remove the tumour, and received radiotherapy and chemotherapy. Jane is a very active person, and a public figure with a high profile. She often works late into the night, and is often away travelling to conferences and meetings. She tried to carry on working as normal during her cancer treatment. Jane finds it very hard to stop thinking about work, and often cannot switch off, which makes it hard for her to go to sleep. She often has severe hot flushes, which started with the menopause, and were exacerbated by the radiotherapy. She is always thirsty, with a dry mouth. When she came to see me she was suffering from severe anxiety and feelings of panic.

In terms of Chinese medicine, the background to her cancer is yin deficiency. By over-working, and not allowing her body to rest, she has exhausted her yin. This has caused her to be undernourished, overheated and dried out. We can note that her cancer occurred in the upper body, which tends to be more yin deficient, that is more hot and dry. Yin allows us to "switch off", and when we are switched off our bodies can repair and renew themselves. By never entering into that yin state of relaxation, the body and mind had become exhausted. This had allowed the cancer to develop.

Acupuncture was very effective in helping Jane to switch off, and she would often fall asleep on the treatment couch. After a course of twenty sessions, she had become able to switch off from work and to go to sleep more easily. She felt much less anxiety, and was not experiencing any sensations of panic. The acupuncture had considerably eased the facial pain she had experienced following surgery, to the extent that she did not need painkillers.

A SUMMARY OF EXCESS AND DEFICIENCY

- An *excess* pattern is one where something is there that should not be there.

- A tumour itself is an *excess* by definition.

- The main *excess* patterns seen in cancer tumours are phlegm and blood stagnation.

- Conventional medicine can be very good at getting rid of the tumour itself (the *excess* part of the disease).

- Underlying most cancers are patterns of *deficiency*.

- The most common pattern is *qi deficiency*.

- Often there is also *deficiency* of blood, yin and yang.

- Conventional medicine usually does not attempt to address the *deficiency* aspect of cancer, which is where Chinese medicine is very useful.

- Side effects of conventional cancer treatments can cause deficiencies. This is by no means to say that one should not receive conventional treatments, rather that one should address their side effects with Chinese medicine.

External (yang) and internal (yin)

In Chinese medicine, cancer is an internal condition by definition, so we do need to spend time diagnosing whether it is internal or external. Certain factors contributing to the cancer may initially have been external, such as pollution or viruses, but by the time the cancer has developed it is classed as internal.

Summary of Eight Principles diagnosis

The "Eight Principles" model is the cornerstone of Chinese medicine. It allows us to organise complex patterns of information into a coherent picture. Although in essence it is a simple system, its combinations are infinite. Each person has a unique diagnostic picture, and so the Eight Principles captures something of the wonderful complexities of the human being. It is well worth referring back to this section as you read the book, because each time you revisit the Eight Principles you will grasp it in greater depth.

One must have an accurate Eight Principles diagnosis before any treatment is given. All of the techniques and advice in this book are based on the Eight Principles. If at all possible, one should obtain a diagnosis from an experienced practitioner of Chinese medicine in order to get the most from this book.

THE CHINESE ORGAN SYSTEM

The first point to make about the Chinese organs is that they are understood in quite a different way than the orthodox western organs. Whereas western medicine sees the organs primarily as *physical objects*, Chinese medicine sees them also as *functional systems*. The organs have both physical properties, and energetic properties. We can draw an analogy with our understanding of light, which can be understood as both physical particles and energy.

In fact, we should not really translate the Chinese organs directly into western organs at all. Westerners have done this, because that is how we think. We see the body as discreet lumps of physical matter, so that is how we have translated Chinese medicine. The Chinese tended to go along with these translations, because they gave credibility to Chinese medicine as "scientific". But in fact the essence of Chinese medicine is distorted by translating Chinese medical terms directly into western terms.

For example, the Chinese character "gan" is translated as "liver". The original character "gan" actually implies a system of sluice gates, which control the flow of water in irrigated fields (much of Chinese medicine derives from the agricultural systems being developed at the time). If the gan were not working properly, some fields would be flooded, and others parched. Similarly, in the human person, the gan regulates the flow of substances through the whole body. It can be thought of as the gate in each cell, regulating the flow of nutrients in, and waste out. If the gan is not working properly, there will be stagnation of substances such as blood and food. The gan also regulates the flow of qi, and if the qi stagnates, the person will feel irritable or angry.

So, we can see that in translating "gan" with the word "liver" we miss the whole point of Chinese medicine. Gan is a concept involving mind and body, a system which pervades the *whole person*. When those trained in western medicine study Chinese medicine, and are told that the liver "regulates qi", their immediate response is usually "but the liver does not do that!". So when reading this book, please always bear this in mind. For now, Chinese medicine is still taught using terms such as "liver", although some Chinese doctors feel that one should use the Chinese terms instead.

Because the organs are not just localised lumps of matter, they can not be understood in isolation from each other. In Chinese medicine the *interaction* of the organs is very important. The organs work very closely together, and disharmony in one organ will bring disharmony in the others. Cancer in one area will necessarily involve imbalances in other parts. An advanced pathology such as cancer is a *systemic* disease, involving the whole system: to simply cut it out is not enough.

Chinese medicine recognises five organs as the most important ones, and we shall look at each of these in turn.

The digestive system[5]

The Chinese character for this is "pi", which implies a servant. If the servant is good, he will cook the food well, transport it to the master on time, and clear away the leftovers efficiently. If the servant is lazy, he will cause much sickness and distress to the master. The master will be too worried about the mess to concentrate on higher matters. The quality of the servant is one of the key determinants of health.

Like every organ, the digestive system has its own kind of qi, which we call "digestive qi".[6] The key function of the digestive qi is to transform food into blood and qi, in other words to extract nutrients and energy from food (remember that one function of qi is to transform). When a person has strong digestive qi (a good servant), they extract nutrients efficiently. However, when they have weak digestive qi, they will struggle to break their food down and absorb it: the undigested food will turn into phlegm. *Weak digestive qi is the main cause of phlegm in the body.* Phlegm can form tumours, so one key aspect of working with cancer is to strengthen the digestive qi.

From a western perspective, weak digestive qi corresponds to problems such as a lack of digestive enzymes, bloating, weight gain, malabsorption, food intolerances, and problems with peristalsis (the rhythmic contractions of the muscles around the gut

---

5   Most textbooks of Chinese medicine translate this with the word "spleen". This is a bad translation which has caused much misunderstanding among students and patients.

6   Known as "spleen qi" in Chinese medical textbooks.

which push food through the digestive tract). Because these people have problems turning food into energy, they will often crave sweet foods, because these foods contain sugars which are more easily transformed into energy. The problem is that a diet which is high in sugar has been found to be a contributory factor in certain cancers.

When a person is not extracting the energy from his food, he will feel tired. If this situation continues over a long period of time, the person may become chronically fatigued. There will be a general qi deficiency, which may contribute to the development of cancer.

Weak digestive qi can contribute to many kinds of cancers, as it leads to general qi deficiency, and to the build up of phlegm. It is particularly relevant to stomach cancer, colo-rectal cancer, and all phlegm types of cancer.

As we have explained, the organs have a mental aspect too. We shall see later in the book that digestive problems can be associated with worry, or "over-thinking".

The liver

The Chinese character "gan", which is translated as "liver", actually implies a gate, which regulates the flow of substances through the body.

If the gate system is not working properly, we call this pathology *liver qi stagnation*. This may in turn lead to *blood stagnation*, which as we saw in the above section on the Four Fullnesses can be a major contributory factor in many kinds of cancers. The major cause of blood stagnation is liver qi stagnation. It is therefore essential in working with cancer to ensure the smooth flow of liver qi.

On a cellular level, the liver promotes the smooth movement of nutrients into cells, and the removal of waste products. Liver qi stagnation can therefore cause a build up of toxins in the cells. This can create inflammatory conditions such as colitis (inflammation of the colon). In Chinese medicine we call this situation a build up of *heat toxins*. These toxins prevent the cells from working efficiently, allowing the formation of tumours.

Qi flows through channels, called meridians, into each organ. The liver meridian runs through the breast area, so *liver qi stagnation* is often a major contributory factor in breast cancer. The liver meridian also flows into the uterus and genitals, and stagnation can also contribute to cancers in these areas.

The digestive qi *produces* the blood, but it is the liver which *stores* the blood. Rather than talking of general blood deficiency, to be more accurate we should refer to *liver blood deficiency*.

It is recognised in western medicine that chemotherapy can have an adverse effect on the liver function. It can cause certain liver enzymes to be raised, as the liver struggles to deal with the toxic effects of the chemicals. According to Chinese medicine, this can contribute to liver blood deficiency.

We shall see later in the book that liver pathologies can be associated with a lack of creativity and anger.

The kidneys

As with the Chinese "liver", the Chinese "kidneys" are quite different from the western kidneys. The key function of the Chinese kidneys is to store the "essence" (in Chinese "jing"). The essence is a kind of reservoir of energy, which nourishes the other organs. We can think of the essence as the constitution of the person. The quality of essence determines the general health and vitality of the person.

We can also think of the essence as the genetic make up of the individual. Someone who has a strong gene pool could be said to have strong essence. The essence is also responsible for reproduction. This is true both in terms of producing children, and in terms of cellular reproduction. In terms of children, the stronger the essence, the stronger the offspring. In cellular terms, the stronger the essence, the more accurately cells will reproduce. If the essence is weak, the cells are more likely to mutate. Some of these mutations may be cancerous.

According to Chinese medicine it is very hard to increase the amount of essence a person has. Emphasis is therefore placed on *preserving* the essence, and we shall see how to do this in later chapters.

We can break down the essence into its yin part and its yang part. The essence can be conceived as a reservoir of yin, and a reservoir of yang. The kidneys are therefore known as the source of all yin and yang in the body.

We can think of qi as the body's *current* bank account, and essence as the body's *savings* account. Qi is earnt, and then spent. If we earn more than we spend, we can save. In other words, if we produce more qi than we use, we can save the surplus as essence. If we are careful in our lives to look after ourselves, if we eat well and rest properly, we can preserve our essence. On the other hand, if we use up our qi faster than we produce it, if we "burn the candle at both ends", we need to spend our savings, and we deplete our essence. If this situation continues, we risk spending all our savings, and becoming bankrupt. When the essence gets low, we are "running on empty". We cannot cope with stress, we cannot recover from illness, and we feel constantly exhausted. We call this situation *kidney essence deficiency*. In this situation, both the kidney yin and the kidney yang are exhausted.

We can think of parts of the hormonal system as coming under the Chinese kidney system. The Chinese kidneys are responsible for setting the base metabolism of the body, so we can think of the thyroid gland as part of the Chinese kidney system. If the thyroid is *under-active*, the base metabolism is too low, and the person has all the signs of *kidney yang deficiency:* tiredness, weight gain, coldness and sluggishness. If the thyroid is *over-active*, the base metabolism is too high, and the person has all the signs of *kidney yin deficiency:* restlessness, insomnia and overheating.

We can also think of the balance between adrenaline and serotonin in terms of the balance between kidney yang and kidney yin respectively. Adrenaline allows us to move into the "fight or flight" mode, so we can think of it as part of the kidney yang, allowing us to be active and stimulated. Serotonin, on the other hand, allows us to switch into relaxation, rest and repair mode, so we can think of it as part of the kidney yin function. When yin and yang are "harmonised", we can produce adrenaline or serotonin as appropriate. When yin and yang are "out of balance", we are unable to relax, but also unable to get started.

The Chinese liver and kidneys together can be thought of as responsible for the hormonal system as a whole.

We shall see in the chapter on cultivating the spirit that kidney problems may be caused by fear or anxiety. They can be helped by cultivating a sense of stillness.

The lungs

The Chinese lungs have a much wider meaning than just the physical organs. The lungs are our interface between us and the outside world, and form our boundaries. If we have strong lung qi, we can take in what we need, and exclude the rest. This is true on both the physical and mental levels. On the physical level, the lungs form a boundary between us and whatever surrounds us. They allow us to take in "good qi" (including oxygen, in western terms), and help us to expel "bad qi", such as pollution and viruses.

The lungs also function on the mental/emotional level. They allow us to absorb positive emotions, while keeping out too much negative emotion. If our lung qi is weak, we easily absorb other people's negative feelings, to the extent that we feel drained by them. I have worked with many cancer patients who became ill after looking after very sick people for long periods of time, both personally and professionally. We must work to strengthen the lungs to give us good boundaries with other people. With strong lung qi, one can be compassionate without feeling drained.

The Chinese lungs govern what we would call the immune system, and this is why they are very important in working with cancer. If the immune system is strong, it will fight cancer cells as soon as they start to appear, and destroy them. In fact, we all have cancer cells inside us all of the time, but our immune system is usually effective enough to kill them before they develop. We will see in the section on herbal medicine that some Chinese herbs which have traditionally been used to strengthen the lungs have recently been found to promote the production of certain immune cells which are active against cancer cells.

The Chinese lungs are said to have a *dispersing* function. This means that they should disperse any accumulation in the chest area, such as phlegm, or stagnant qi. When the lung qi is weak, phlegm can build up in the chest, and qi can stagnate there. This can contribute to the formation of tumours in the chest, such as lung and breast cancers.

The lungs are also said to govern the skin, indeed it is said that the skin is the third lung. Like the lung organ, the skin forms a boundary between us and the outside world. Some kinds of skin cancer are therefore associated with the lungs in Chinese medicine.

The lungs are affected by grief. I have certainly treated a number of patients who developed lung or breast cancer following the death of a loved one.

If a person has weak lungs, we say that they have *lung qi deficiency.*

The heart

As with western medicine, the Chinese heart is responsible for the flow of blood around the body. However, the Chinese heart is also known as the *seat of the emotions,* as it used to be in the West. Indeed, in English we have many phrases which remind us of the fuller understanding of the heart which we once had. We talk of speaking from the heart, of loving someone with all our heart, of wearing our heart on our sleeves. This used to be much more than figurative language, as one can see from looking at the history of European medicine, which traditionally understood the heart to play a prominent role in the personality.

In Chinese medicine the heart is also the place where the "spirit" resides. Indeed, many religious traditions share the Chinese understanding that the heart is our connection with the Divine. In the Orthodox Christian Church the heart is recognised as the *organ of spiritual perception,* and great emphasis is placed on using the "Prayer of the Heart" to approach God. St Isaac the Syrian said that "God secretes Himself into the human heart". We shall look at this whole area more fully in the chapter on cultivating the spirit. Suffice for now to say that the state of the person's heart has a profound impact on their well-being.

In Chinese medicine we say that the heart tends to overheat. This overheating is often caused by emotional problems, which can be exacerbated by receiving a cancer diagnosis. Because of their "hot" nature, chemotherapy and radiotherapy can also heat up the heart.

If the heart is overheated for a long period of time, the heat dries out the heart yin, causing *heart yin deficiency.* The symptoms of heart yin deficiency can include severe anxiety, panic, insomnia, intense feelings of heat, and palpitations.

We have already mentioned liver blood deficiency. This syndrome can lead on to *heart blood deficiency*. The symptoms of this condition are similar to heart yin deficiency, but there is less overheating.

A summary of the main organ pathologies involved in cancer

DIGESTIVE SYSTEM

- Digestive qi deficiency (weak digestive system, tendency to worry).

- Phlegm (certain kinds of tumours).

LIVER

- Liver qi stagnation (inadequate movement of substances in the body, feelings of "stuckness" or anger).

- Liver blood deficiency (nutritional deficiencies).

- Blood stagnation (certain kinds of tumours).

- Heat toxins (presence of certain chemicals which may encourage the formation of tumours).

KIDNEYS

- Kidney yin deficiency (lack of rest and repair, overheating, inability to relax, fear, restlessness).

- Kidney yang deficiency (lack of movement, coldness, stagnation, inability to "get going", lack of motivation, fear).

- Kidney essence deficiency (kidney yin deficiency and kidney yang deficiency together).

LUNGS

- Lung qi deficiency (weak immune system, breathing problems, lack of boundaries, grief).

HEART

- Heart yin deficiency (emotional problems with heat).

- Heart blood deficiency (emotional problems with no heat signs).

Case history showing organ interactions: Mary, aged 42

Constitutionally, Mary had always had weak kidney energy. Puberty came late for her, and her cycle was always erratic (the Chinese kidneys govern reproduction and development). She had problems conceiving, but eventually had a baby girl. She had always suffered from tiredness, but following the birth she suffered from complete exhaustion. She started to have digestive problems at this time, as the kidneys were not able to give proper support to the digestive qi. She began to feel increasingly unable to cope with life, and this placed a great deal of stress on her. The stress started to affect her liver, and she began to experience uncontrollable outbursts of rage at those around her, especially pre-menstrually. Her period cycle had become more erratic than ever. She was suffering from "liver qi stagnation". Mary started to put on a lot of weight, partly as she was too tired to exercise properly, and partly because she could not break down her food due to her digestive weakness. In other words, she began to accumulate "phlegm". She started to "comfort eat" to try and give herself more energy, and to make herself feel better, but this led to further weight increases, low self-esteem and depression. The depression caused the liver qi to stagnate still further, and caused the lung qi to stagnate too. One day she felt a lump in her left breast, which was diagnosed as cancer.

In this case we see how four organs are involved in creating a serious imbalance in the whole person. There is not one cause of the cancer, rather there is a pattern of disharmony. The pattern involves both physical and mental factors. In the other chapters of the book we shall see how Chinese medicine can help to address this kind of pattern.

Summary of the Chinese organ system

The Chinese organs are conceived as dynamic, energetic, functional systems, which are not limited to the physical dimension. Rather, they encompass the mental–emotional state of the person. Through understanding the Chinese organ system, we can begin to see how the physical and mental aspects of the human person are intimately related. *Illness usually arises because of disharmonies at both the physical and mental levels.*

The Chinese organs are never considered in isolation, but always seen in the context of the other organs, and of the whole system. Cancer is never just a *local* problem, but is always seen as a disharmony of the *whole system.*

In the rest of the book, we shall examine in more depth some of the factors which contribute to the development of imbalances in the organs, and which can lead to cancer. By gaining a deeper understanding of these imbalances, we can begin to correct them, and to return towards harmony.

THE FIVE ELEMENTS

According to the ancient Chinese view of the universe, everything was thought to be composed of five elements. These elements were held to be the building blocks of the whole universe. All things were thought to be composed of the elements in different proportions, and the exact mix of the elements gives each substance its individual properties. This idea was very similar to the ancient Greek idea of the elements, which was developed around the same time as the Chinese system, and which formed the basis of western medicine until around the 17th century.

According to the elemental theory, the human person is formed of the same elements as the rest of creation. When these elements are in the correct proportion, the person is in harmony and health. When one element is deficient, or in excess, the person becomes ill.

According to the Greek view, there were four elements: water, fire, earth and air. According to the Chinese view, there were five elements: water, fire, earth, metal and wood. The systems are very similar, but the properties of the elements are arranged differently.

Of course, we now know that there are around 100 "elements" in a chemical sense, not just four or five. Rather than thinking of the five elements in literal, physical terms, we can think of them as archetypes. If the five archetypes are present in good proportions, the person will be healthy. If any one element is over-dominant or lacking, the person will tend to fall sick. The five elements model helps us see that true health is based on balance between various factors. For example, there

The Five Elements correspondences

	Water	Wood	Fire	Earth	Metal
Colour	Black/ blue	Green	Red	Yellow	White
Season	Winter	Spring	Summer	Late summer	Autumn
Climate disliked	Cold	Wind	Heat	Damp	Dryness
Main organ	Kidneys	Liver	Heart	Digestive system ("Spleen")	Lungs
Secondary organ	Bladder	Gall bladder	Small intestine	Stomach	Colon
Tissue governed	Bone	Tendons/ joints	Blood vessels	Muscles/ flesh	Skin
Sense organ	Ears	Eyes	Tongue (speech)	Tongue (taste)	Nose
Emotion	Fear	Anger	Joy	Worry	Grief
Voice	Groaning	Shouting	Laughing	Singing	Weeping
Taste	Salty	Sour	Bitter	Sweet	Spicy
Smell	Putrid	Rancid	Burnt	Fragrant	Acrid
Mental aspect	Willpower	Imagination/ creativity	Spirit/ heart– mind	Intellect	"Earthly soul"

must be structure (metal), but also flexibility (wood); there must be expansion (fire), but also contraction (water); and there must be a centre holding it all together (earth).

Likewise, the year is made up of seasons, which should exist in certain proportions to give a balanced climate. Too much global warming is not good.

We can use an orchestra as an analogy: to get a harmonious sound we need a balance between the various instruments. None should be too loud, and none too soft. The instruments should take turns to shine, then make way for the others. The instruments must be in tune with each other.

Or we can think of pure white light, which is composed of the correct balance between the seven colours. If any colour is over-or under-dominant the light will not be pure white. It will not be *whole*.

As we go through the book, we shall see how this works in more detail. The task of the practitioner is to identify which elements are out of balance, and to try and correct them.

The Five Elements correspondences help one to identify which organ is most out of balance. If a person has either a craving or an aversion to the correspondences of a certain element, it is likely that the organ of that element is the cause of illness. Let us say that a person always wears green, loves the springtime, hates wind, has problems with their joints and eyes, has a tendency to shout and be angry, and is a frustrated artist (that is, they have not developed their creative talents as they would wish). It is very likely that this person has a liver imbalance.

The beauty of this system is that once one has identified the organ which is out of balance, a whole range of advice automatically follows. Our frustrated artist must find ways to channel his anger, and spend more time being creative. He should ensure he does not over-indulge in sour food, but has enough. If possible he could move to a less windy climate, or at least avoid exposure to the wind.

As we shall see throughout the book, this system is used in many ways by Chinese medicine. It is used to select the appropriate food and herbs, as we shall see in those chapters. Each taste has an energetic quality associated with it, which can be used to treat the relevant organ. For example, the bitter taste (fire) clears heat, and so benefits the heart (the fire organ), which dislikes heat. The sweet taste (earth) tonifies, so supports a weak digestive system (the earth organ).

We shall see in the chapter on cultivating the spirit that developing the mental and emotional aspects of an element can have profound effects on the physical organs.

We shall see in the chapter on qi cultivation that environmental influences can have a great influence on the organs, through the elements system.

The five elements is a truly holistic system. It examines all influences on a person, and attempts to ensure that these influences contribute to a harmonious pattern. This system shows us what a profound impact diet, lifestyle, mental state and environment have on us. Disharmony in any of the areas we have discussed can bring illness. But *knowledge of the elements can help to restore harmony.*

THE CAUSES OF DISEASE

The Chinese medical model, which we still use today, was developed around the same time as the ancient Greek model was used by Hippocrates and his contemporaries. The two systems have much in common. Both systems were, at that time, in the process of changing how they understood the causes of disease. Previously, great emphasis had been placed on the role of the supernatural in the cause of disease, in particular the role of "evil spirits". In both China and the Greek world, this view was gradually being replaced by the view that disease was caused primarily by *natural* factors, rather than supernatural ones. These factors included:

- diet

- emotions

- climate
- poisons/toxins
- other lifestyle factors
- constitution.

Let's look at the Chinese understanding of each factor.

Diet

It was believed that the energetic properties of food had a profound influence. Consuming too many foods which were "hot" (energetically speaking) would cause the person to become too hot, for example. "Hot" foods include certain spices, fried foods, and red meat, as well as alcohol. These would cause the kind of hot symptoms we mentioned above. Other foods tend to cause phlegm, such as dairy products, wheat and sugar.

Emotions

The psycho-emotional state of the person has a great impact on the physical body. In Chinese medicine, each organ is harmed by a particular emotion. Anger harms the liver, grief harms the lungs, and so on. Suffice to say for now that this insight is certainly confirmed by modern research, which has shown that the emotions influence the hormonal system, and that in turn the hormonal system influences the body.

Climate

It was observed in ancient China that certain diseases occurred in particular climates. This was formalised into a system whereby each organ was understood to be harmed by a specific climate.

Damp harms the digestive system, cold harms the kidneys, and so on. This area will be looked at in the chapter on qi cultivation.

Poisons/toxins

Chinese medicine recognised the role of poisons, as well as "external pathogens". These "pathogens" were basically microorganisms, such as viruses and bacteria. As well as attempting to expel any pathogens present, it was also considered important to strengthen the immune system of the patient. Again, modern research is confirming the importance of the immune system in fighting cancer.

Other lifestyle factors

It was recognised that, for men, excessive sex could weaken the body, by depleting the "essence". For women, having too many children could do the same thing. Too much physical work could also deplete the essence, whereas a lack of exercise could cause the qi to stagnate. Thus, the Chinese advised moderation in all things.

Constitution

The ancient Chinese were well aware that the health of the parents had a profound impact on the health of the children. This was particularly true of the mother, who influences the child not only by her constitution, but also by providing the environment in which the foetus grows. It was recognised that weakness in specific organs could be inherited, which today we would understand as genetic inheritance. Chinese medicine always seeks to improve the underlying constitution of the patient.

TONGUE DIAGNOSIS

In Chinese medicine, the appearance of the tongue gives much detailed information about the internal condition of the patient. We can look at several aspects of tongue diagnosis in turn.

The shape of the tongue

A swollen tongue indicates general qi deficiency. This is because the qi moves fluids, and when the qi is weak the fluids accumulate, causing damp and phlegm. The swollen tongue indicates that there is damp and phlegm in the body. A swollen tongue is often seen in patients whose cancer is of the phlegm type.

A flat tongue indicates liver blood deficiency. A flat tongue is an undernourished tongue, and this indicates an undernourished body. Often radiotherapy causes a flat tongue, as it is said to dry the blood.

The colour of the tongue body

- A normal tongue should be pink.

- A red tongue body indicates that heat is present in the patient. Chemotherapy and radiotherapy often cause the tongue body to be red.

- A pale tongue indicates deficiency. A pale, *moist* tongue indicates *qi* deficiency. A pale *dry* tongue indicates *blood* deficiency.

- A purple tongue indicates blood stagnation, which is a key factor in many types of cancer.

The colour of the tongue coat

A normal tongue should have a thin white coat. A thick white coat usually indicates phlegm. A thick yellow coat indicates *hot* phlegm.

Other features

Cracks indicate yin deficiency. A cracked tongue is like parched earth, which cracks due to lack of moisture and nourishment. Radiotherapy and chemotherapy often cause a cracked tongue, as their heating effects dry out the yin.

Lumps on the tongue indicate an advanced state of congestion and stagnation. They are often seen in those with cancer.

The areas of the tongue

Each organ is represented by a specific area of the tongue. If one sees the above features in one of these areas, this indicates a problem in that area. For example, if only the heart area of the tongue was red, this would indicate heat in the heart.

Different parts of the tongue correspond to different organs as follows:

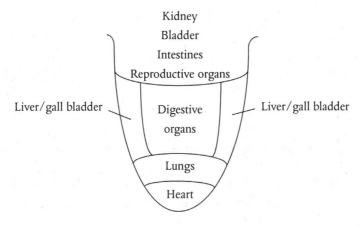

Kidney

Bladder

Intestines

Reproductive organs

Liver/gall bladder

Digestive organs

Liver/gall bladder

Lungs

Heart

PULSE DIAGNOSIS

Detailed pulse diagnosis is way beyond the scope of this book, and takes many years to master. The practitioner of Chinese medicine will spend a long time listening to the quality of the pulse, not just its timing.

One listens to the pulse to determine whether it feels too "full" or too "empty". A pulse which feels very full indicates an *excess* condition, such as phlegm or blood stagnation. A pulse which is hard to find, or which feels very weak, indicates a *deficiency* condition.

A rapid pulse indicates heat in the body, while a slow pulse indicates cold (unless the person is extremely fit, in which case a slow pulse is normal).

The timing of the pulse is also important: a normal pulse should beat nice and steadily. If the strength of the pulse varies while it is being taken, this indicates *qi stagnation*. If the variation is very marked, this suggests *blood stagnation*.

If the pulse varies in timing, that is if it speeds up and slows down while being taken, this indicates *qi stagnation*. If the variation is marked, this suggests *blood stagnation*.

The pulse positions are as follows:

Pulse positions

Wrist	
Right (qi side)	**Left** (blood side)
Lungs	Heart
Spleen	Liver
Kidney yang	Kidney yin

There are three pulse positions at each wrist, each corresponding to one organ. We take the pulse at both wrists, giving a total of six positions in all. There is one position for each of the five organs we have studied, except for the kidneys which have two positions.

The pulse changes when acupuncture needles are inserted. Many practitioners monitor the pulse change to ensure the treatment is having the desired effect.

SUMMARY

Chinese medicine offers a detailed and profound understanding of the human person, and what makes us well. We shall find as we go through this book that these insights are increasingly backed up by modern research. Chinese medicine shows us that the human person is a complex entity, composed of many inter-related strands. The person is intimately connected to his surroundings. Disease is not usually caused by one thing only, but by a *pattern* of factors. This is particularly true of a complex pathology such as cancer.

This means that medical intervention must be complex. It is never enough to apply one technique in isolation, and it is always important to educate the patient regarding lifestyle factors. We shall see that this makes it hard to use modern research methods to evaluate Chinese medicine. Modern research methods specifically try to measure *one* variable at a time, and keep all the others constant, in order to monitor the impact of the changing variable. While we welcome wholeheartedly modern research into Chinese medicine, we must always bear this point in mind. The traditional Chinese approach to cancer is to try and use *all* methods possible to give the patient the best chance of beating the disease, and the best chance of improving quality of life.

CHAPTER TWO

Cultivating the Spirit: The Psychology of Chinese Medicine

CHAPTER CONTENTS

INTRODUCTION

By the time the *Yellow Emperor* was collated, in the two centuries BC, the theories underpinning Chinese medicine had become fairly well developed. These theories drew on the general philosophical ideas which had been around for the few hundred years beforehand. In this chapter, we shall explore some of those ideas, and show how they can be used to enrich the experience of Chinese medicine.

The idea was prevalent that self-cultivation was the highest form of medicine, if the hardest to master. By cultivating the self, it was thought that one became more whole, and that this brought physical health benefits too.

The *Yellow Emperor* harked back to a time when people lived in harmony with the Tao, and were healthier because of it.

Somehow people had fallen away from this state of harmony, and the idea arose that one could attempt to recapture it. Thus the idea of "cultivating the Tao" arose. This consisted of living a more simple, natural way of life. In addition, special importance was placed on cultivating the mind. By aligning one's mind to the Tao, one could return to the state of harmony enjoyed by the ancients.

What is Tao? There is no direct translation into English. The word can mean "way", or "path", in the sense of a path to wholeness, harmony or truth. The word can also mean the natural order of things, or the "natural law" of the cosmos. Each thing has its own nature, its own particular way of being. If all things are allowed to exist according to their own nature, harmony will prevail. Conversely, if man attempts to "improve" things, to go against the natural order, against Tao, disharmony will result.

According to some, Tao has metaphysical implications, and implies the Divine Organising Principle of the Universe. It transcends time and space, pre-existing the birth of the universe. It is also the "mother" of all things, the source of all being. However, others do not stress this aspect, and see Tao primarily as a more "natural" way of being. In any case, Tao is undefinable by words, and beyond comprehension.

As the word "Tao" is open to many interpretations, we can say that it is by no means incompatible with any religion. Indeed, Chinese medicine has been practised for over two millennia by people of all religions. In modern atheist China, the Taoist aspect of Chinese medicine is greatly downplayed. Indeed, in the Cultural Revolution Taoism was judged to be incompatible with an atheist worldview. However, many would argue that the practice of Chinese medicine in modern China lacks a certain dimension because of its purely secular approach. Certainly, the psycho-emotional aspects of illness tend to be greatly downplayed.

This chapter will look at the natural philosophies behind Chinese medicine. In other words, philosophies of how man relates to the natural world. We will also look at the psychological/emotional aspects of Chinese medicine, in other words at how it relates to the mind. We can draw a distinction between this approach, and an approach which seeks to make Chinese medicine a kind of quasi religion, or a supernatural practice. For this author, Chinese medicine is a *natural* medicine, which can be practised by people of any religion or of none. Its aim is to bring us into harmony with the laws of nature, not to transcend those laws.

It is certainly true that "Taoism" later became a religion, with priests, doctrines, and certain ascetic practices, involving "internal alchemy". However, the thinkers who inspired "Taoism" were not "Taoists", they were free thinkers, and did not set out to form a religion, or an "ism". One doubts very much whether they were "Taoists"!

THE FIVE ELEMENTS

In Chapter One, we introduced the idea that the universe is composed of five elements. The mind is one with the universe, and is therefore also composed of these elements. We can think of these elements as *psychological aspects* of the mind. When these five areas are well developed, the personality is more rounded and complete. Just as nature, Tao, is composed of a harmonious relationship between the elements, so should the human mind be.

Water

Water governs that part of the mind known as the "zhi" in Chinese. Zhi can be translated as willpower, and governs our motivation, and fundamental direction in life. If we have a strong zhi, we will be highly motivated, with a strong sense of purpose. If we have weak zhi, we will lack direction and motivation, and will drift through life. The zhi is symbolised as a turtle, or tortoise, which moves slowly, but with a steady purpose. Because it does not waste energy rushing around, the tortoise lives a very long time. This teaches us that to achieve our goal, we must not be "busy", but must be constant. In the fable about the tortoise and the hare, the hare rushes off ahead, but the tortoise wins because he has a sense of purpose, and moves forward slowly and steadily. In our society, we tend to be very "busy", but what is all this busyness achieving? Is it bringing us nearer our true goal?

Water is connected with death and rebirth, in the sense of old ideas dying and new ones being born. Often, people with cancer feel that it has given them a chance to grow and change, to see things in a new light. The possible approach of death gives life a new perspective. Instead of ploughing on as if through an endless tunnel, suddenly each day, each moment, can seem very precious. Some of my patients have said that they try to live each day as if it may be their last, which can bring immense joy and release.

Water also means purification, and getting rid of surplus baggage. Cancer can be an opportunity to shed what is no longer needed, to focus on what matters, which is often love. Attitudes such as jealousy, material possessiveness, and competitiveness, are seen for what they are: a futile waste of energy. When one's lifespan may be short, one no longer has time to waste. Old "friends" may fall away, and deeper bonds may be formed with those that remain.

For many, water is about taking a step back from the everyday world, with its concerns for money and status. It is about examining one's fundamental motivation in life. It is like a hamster suddenly getting off the treadmill, and asking why he had been on it all these years. Rather than working hard to go round in circles, water is about finding one's direction. When one has found it, one becomes persistent, like water wearing down a rock.

Water is about stopping the struggle, and "going with the flow". Instead of fighting everything and everyone, it teaches acceptance. One learns to wait until the time is right, to ride the wave. One watches where the current is going and swims with it, rather than trying to swim upstream. People with cancer are often worn down by the fight, and it can come as a great relief to discover that it is all right not to struggle. Sometimes it is good to surrender, to rest.

Water is about more than just rest, it is about hibernation, about switching off. It is about finding a place of stillness and silence. From this place, one can emerge a richer person.

Water always flows down to the lowest level, and therefore symbolises humility. As Lao Tsu said: "it flows in places men reject and so is like the Tao" (v.8). Sometimes people with cancer feel ashamed, almost as though they got cancer because they deserved it. This idea can come from misguided "spirituality", which says that physical illness reflects spiritual malaise, or that it is a punishment for evil done in this life or a previous one. This idea is simply not true: people with cancer do not deserve it any more than the rest of us. Indeed, some holy people have been given cancer to give them an opportunity to learn something. For example, cancer can teach humility: it is quite hard to be proud with cancer.

The water element, and its organ the kidneys, are associated with fear. Often cancer brings a fear of death. Paradoxically, fear of death can be lessened by cultivating a "fear" of the Tao. More accurately, we can talk about recovering a sense of *awe* at the mystery of creation. This sense of awe is an essential part of our psychology, and we are not whole humans without it.

As Lao Tsu said: "When men lack a sense of awe there will be disaster" (v.72, *Tao Te Ching*, see Further Reading at the end of this chapter). When we live without this sense of reverence, part of us is missing, and things will go wrong.

Instead of a pathological fear, one should cultivate a kind of watchfulness. Confucius said that:

> the sage is watchful and pays attention even when he sees nothing that might call for his vigilance. He is afraid and trembles even when he hears nothing that should frighten him. For him the most important discovery is the secret enfolded by his heart…thus he watches carefully over that which he alone knows.[7]

By this careful watching, and by reflection on the inner life, one avoids pathological, irrational fear. This latter kind of fear is like paranoia, like a man in fear of being arrested. When one is in this state, the thoughts flitter about like tiny birds, unable to rest. On the other hand, if one is watchful and observant, the thoughts settle and become harmonious. Claude Larre, a Jesuit translator and commentator on Chinese medicine, said that, "St Francis of Assisi calling the birds by his very way of being is an example of that".[8]

When the thoughts are unsettled, there is no way for you to know yourself. Finally you will lose the ability to *be* yourself. I have often observed this in people who have just had a diagnosis of cancer, who have been thrown completely out of themselves.

The Yellow Emperor tells us that when a person is dominated by the pathological kind of fear, the qi becomes stagnant. It fails to raise the fluids properly, causing accumulation of damp and phlegm in the lower body, which may contribute to the formation of lumps there.

---

7 From Confucius' "The Doctrine of the Mean", quoted in Larre *The Seven Emotions*, p.92.

8 ibid, p.100.

Wood

Wood governs the part of the personality called the "hun". The hun is concerned with going beyond the mundane, with seeing the "big picture". It is that part of us which seeks to break out of normal routine, to explore new avenues. The hun is symbolised by a dragon, which soars above the mere trees to see the wood. The dragon is a mythical animal, which flies to "other worlds". Similarly, the hun is concerned with the non-material world, and is the part of us which looks to the next world. Depending on one's beliefs, cancer may be an opportunity to prepare for this. Those who die suddenly do not get that chance.

The hun gives us the capacity for dreams, both when asleep and when awake. It gives us great leaps of imagination, and allows new inventions, revolutions and creativity. In our society it is very easy for us to lose sight of this part of ourselves, and to just focus on paying the bills. Our playful, child-like side is all too easily crushed by the pressures of life.

Many people with cancer rediscover a love for creative pursuits, such as music or painting. Because it is a reminder that one's time is limited, it can make us prioritise what we love to do. It can remind one to leave behind the mundane, to step out of one's everyday self. When we do not do this, when we fail to cultivate our creative side, we can develop liver qi stagnation. Liver is the organ associated with wood and the hun. As we have seen, qi stagnation can contribute to the development of cancer.

The Chinese sage Chuang Tsu also spoke eloquently about human creativity. For him, it was a way for the person to strive for unity with the Tao:

A cook was cutting up an ox for Lord Wenhui. Wherever
His hand touched,
His shoulder leaned,

His foot stepped,
His knee nudged,

The flesh would fall away with a swishing sound. Each slice of the cleaver was right in tune, zip zap! He danced in rhythm to "The Mulberry Grove", moved in concert with the strains of "The Managing Chief".

"Ah, wonderful!" said Lord Wenhui, "that skill can attain such heights!"

The cook put down his cleaver and responded, "What your servant loves is the Way, which goes beyond mere skill. When I first began to cut oxen, what I saw was nothing but whole oxen. After three years, I no longer saw whole oxen. Today, I meet the ox with my Soul rather than looking at it with my eyes. My sense organs stop functioning and my spirit moves as it pleases. In accord with the natural grain, I slice at the great crevices, lead the blade through the great cavities. Following its inherent structure, I never encounter the slightest obstacle even where the veins and arteries come together or where the ligaments and tendons join, much less from obvious big bones. A good cook changes his cleaver once a year because he chops. An ordinary cook changes his cleaver once a month because he hacks. Now I've been using my cleaver for nineteen years and have cut up thousands of oxen with it, but the blade is still as fresh as though it had just come from the grindstone. Between the joints there are spaces, but the edge of the blade has no thickness. Since I am inserting something without any thickness into an empty space, there will certainly be lots of room for the blade to play around in. That's why the blade is still as fresh as though it had just come from the grindstone. Nonetheless, whenever I come to a complicated spot and see that it will be difficult to handle, I cautiously restrain myself, focus my vision, and slow my motion. With an imperceptible movement of the cleaver, plop! And the flesh is already separated, like a clump of earth collapsing to the ground. I stand there holding the cleaver in my hand, look all around me with complacent satisfaction, then I wipe off the cleaver and store it away."

"Wonderful!" said Lord Wenhui, "from hearing the words of the cook, I have learned how to nourish life." (see Mair 1994 in Further Reading at the end of this chapter.)

Part of nourishing our creativity lies in developing our relationship with creation. As a society, we seem to have lost our sense of connection to the wonderful creation of which we are part. Part of being a whole person involves cultivating our relationship with the created world, with the ecosystem. Chinese medicine teaches us that if we do not honour creation, we will become ill. This is obviously an issue for society at large, as well as for us as individuals.

Chinese medicine tells us that if our creative energy is not utilised, we may become frustrated and angry. The Chinese character for anger ("nu") consists of a hand holding down a woman, perhaps a slave. It also shows a heart next to the woman, implying she is emotionally affected by the constraint on her. The character implies a kind of repression, with the woman being held against her will. Thus, anger is pictured as arising from a blockage to our spirit, a reaction against something that is preventing us from being ourselves.

The Chinese way, however, is not to express one's anger by shouting at people. This will make the situation worse, and cause the qi to rush around the body improperly. This will affect the functioning of the other organs, which rely on the liver to regulate the flow of qi. In particular, anger prevents the digestive system from working properly, and hinders the absorption of vital nutrients.

Expressing anger will hurt those around us, and may be returned to us later. If we allow ourselves to become angry in a negative way, it scatters our mind, and prevents us thinking clearly. An ancient Chinese treatise on military arts, Sun Zi's *The Art of War*, advises one to "anger the enemy's general in order to scatter his mind".[9] Anger forces us to lose self-control, and become uncentred.

The Chinese way is to utilise the energy which underlies anger in a positive way. This energy is a kind of explosive force, which can be very destructive, or can be harnessed to do something positive. The Chinese character "nu" implies a kind of raising up of something from the ground against the pressure of gravity, against the force of inertia. It implies creation, a new beginning, a birth.

We can check our anger with watchfulness, as mentioned in the section on water. If we catch anger early on, we can often prevent it growing out of hand. It is easier to pull up a small weed than to chop down a large tree.

It is very interesting that anger can prevent acupuncture working. The Yellow Emperor says that if the patient is angry, one should not needle, as "the patient has no possibility to understand or receive the transmission from the point of the needling to the subtle power of his being".[10] This teaches the importance of self-cultivation: without it, Chinese medicine is of limited effect. Chinese medicine does not force, it persuades. When the patient is making too much noise, they are unable to hear the quiet teaching of the needles. Conversely, if one masters the art of watchfulness, one may not need acupuncture.

---

9   *The Art of War*, trans. Cleary, T. Boston, MA: Shambhala 1989.
10   Quoted in Larre, p.85.

Fire

The part of our personality governed by fire is called the "shen", which lives in the heart. Shen can be translated in many ways, and can mean "spirit", or "heart/mind", or "personality". It is the thing that makes each one of us human and unique. The Chinese say that the shen distinguishes us from animals, allowing rational thought and complex language.

The shen also allows us to feel emotions. However, the Chinese way is not to be over-dominated by emotions. One allows emotions to come and go, but keeps them in balance and check. The shen ensures that each emotion is given space, but no one emotion dominates. Cancer often brings strong emotions, and this is natural: the task of the shen is to ensure that no one emotion becomes completely dominant, and suppresses the others.

If the heart is out of balance, one can suffer from anxiety, insomnia, palpitations and panic. These are all symptoms of a "disturbed shen". These problems can be treated with acupuncture and herbs, but if the shen is cultivated, results are much better. We will see how the Chinese philosophers help one to do this.

Like the hun, the shen is represented by a mythical animal, in this case the phoenix. Like the hun, the shen helps us connect with what lies beyond the everyday reality. It allows us to construct philosophies, to make models of the world, by which we can begin to understand and discuss it. My shen is what allows me to have a complex personality, to be a unique person. It is the very centre of my being.

It is only when I have formed an authentic personality that I can form proper relationships with other people. The shen therefore helps us to relate to each other. The warmth of fire allows us to melt barriers, and form bonds with other humans. Cancer can make or break relationships: some "friends" drift away, but with those who remain a deeper, warmer bond may be forged.

In ancient China, human bonds were cultivated through rituals. Drumming rituals were used to unify the hearts of those present. Our society has, for many, lost any meaningful rituals. We will see below that ritual was one of the four virtues recommended by Confucius.

In Chinese medicine, the heart is associated with joy. By this we do not mean excitement, or "fun", which seems to have become the sole purpose of modern existence. We mean peacefulness, connectedness with all around us, and a sense of the harmony of all things. This is why the heart is symbolised by the emperor, who is responsible for peace and harmony in the empire. The emperor was also seen as the connection between the people and the Divine. The heart has this function in each person too, of being our "organ of spiritual perception".[11]

Often with cancer this sense of joy and harmony is lost, as fear and worry take over. When this happens, the qi becomes scattered, and the person loses their sense of meaning and purpose. The person becomes uncentred, and his qi leaks out, instead of flowing along the normal channels. The flow of blood is affected, and one is in danger of blood stagnation. As we have seen, this can contribute to certain cancers, and is the last thing that is needed.

The person's ability to relate to others may also be affected, and relationships may be harmed, at just the time when they are needed most.

---

11 The insight that the heart is the organ of spiritual perception is recognised by many religions. In the Christian Orthodox Church the "prayer of the heart" is a core spiritual practice. It aims to open the heart to God. Many who practise it regularly experience intense sensations in the heart area.

Earth

The earth governs the "yi", which is usually translated as "intellect", although that word does not capture the fullness of the term. The yi allows us to absorb and assimilate, much as the digestive system does. Indeed, earth governs the *physical* digestive system, as well as the ability to digest ideas. Just as the physical digestive system takes complex food, and breaks it down to manageable chunks, so the yi takes the complex world, and breaks it down into manageable concepts. The yi is very active when we are studying: you are using your yi to read this book (I hope!).

The yi allows us to integrate new ideas into our worldview, just as we integrate compounds from food into our physical bodies. It allows us to form connections, to form chains of ideas. From there, we can form an integrated personality, a cohesive centre. The Earth element also represents the centre. If we have a strong yi, we feel centred. We are not blown about by every event, or every emotion. If we are centred, we retain our sense of purpose. Yi can also be translated as purpose.

A diagnosis of cancer is very hard to integrate. It can undermine one's sense of purpose, and leave one feeling very uncentred. One can lose the ability to organise one's thoughts properly, and instead a pattern of "over-thinking", or circular thinking, can develop. One is pushed by *external* events, instead of developing *inner* purpose and plans. One loses the overall picture, and becomes obsessed by small details. These "small thoughts" can grow like weeds in the heart, and prevent it calmly seeing the situation, and coming to terms with it. This is the reason why many Chinese philosophers said "do not think".

This situation depletes the blood and the yin of the heart, and causes the heart to overheat. This can lead to insomnia, palpitations, and feelings of panic and anxiety. Just as ideas are not flowing freely, so the qi of the digestive system also begins to stagnate. The ability to absorb food is reduced, and the person struggles to make enough qi. Eventually the person will become exhausted. The Yellow Emperor describes a situation where the digestive system is no longer able to do its job of turning nutrients into flesh and qi:

> Apprehension and anxiety, worries and preoccupations injure the spirits. When the spirits are injured, under the effect of fear, there is a flowing and overflowing without stopping... The spirits injured under the effect of fear, one loses possession of oneself, well rounded forms become emaciated and the mass of flesh is ravaged. (chapter 8) (see footnote 3, p.17)

One way to counter this situation is to cultivate another earth attribute: contentment. This is a hard lesson, but amidst the turmoil of cancer can one find some contentment with one's life? Can one take pleasure in what one has had from life so far? Can one give thanks for the life enjoyed, rather than focusing on that part of life we may not be granted? Some of my patients have told me that the possible approach of death has made them find more to appreciate in life, more to be contented about. When life seems endless, we take much for granted. When it may be short, we must try to make the most out of each precious day.

Earth represents completion and fulfilment. One of the benefits of cancer over sudden unexpected death is that it gives one a chance to come to terms with life, to draw it to a close. It gives one a chance to *complete* one's life. One can say those things that need to be said. One can apologise and make amends, if needed. One can set one's affairs in order. One can give thanks. One can pull the threads together, and hopefully make one's peace. In other words, one can cultivate reflection and acceptance, rather than being caught up in the small details of life.

Metal

The emotion associated with metal is grief, which is one of the most common emotions associated with cancer. The grief of leaving behind loved ones, and the grief of those left behind. The pain of separation can be unbearable, whatever one's beliefs. There is no way round this pain, we are human beings.

In ancient China, there was a ritual mourning period. This period varied, depending on how close one was to the departed, but lasted several years for close relatives. During this time, one wore solemn clothes, spoke in lowered tones, and refrained from dancing and parties. In other words, people had a chance to grieve properly. They had time to come to terms with the loss of a loved one, without quickly having to put on a cheerful face again. After the official mourning period was over, rituals were still held from time to time for the dead person. As we have said, ritual was one of the four virtues of Confucius, considered essential for a full and harmonious life.

Confucius said that ritual was a guide, something to help us towards an inner transformation. It should never be done in a slavish, empty way. A man whose father had died came to see Confucius, and said that he felt he had finished mourning for his father inside himself, even though the ritual period was not complete. He asked whether Confucius was prepared to exempt him from his official mourning. Confucius replied that yes, of course, there was no point carrying on the ritual in an empty way. After the man left, Confucius broke into tears (which he rarely did), crying at the heart of a man who could get over his father so quickly.

Like the man who went to see Confucius about his father, many in our society do death very quickly. Many would argue that a ritual mourning period would be a constraint on freedom, preferring to leave matters to the individual. However, rituals can *protect* freedom, by shielding people against pressure, and giving them space to grieve properly. When it is the norm to grieve, people feel all right about doing so. When it is the norm to "just get on with it", people feel pressured into doing just that.

This would have been considered very unwise in ancient China, and indeed in many European countries until quite recently. According to the ancient Chinese understanding, one can only move on from an emotion once it has run its natural course. Often, the lack of proper grieving means that people have not let go of the dead person properly, which is not healthy.

Metal is about letting go. Metal is used to make swords, and swords are used to cut. At some point, we have to cut the bond with the dead person. This does not mean we forget them, far from it. As the ancient Chinese did, and as many other cultures still do, it is good to have rituals to remember the dead. However, in some sense one must make that break, and come to terms with the loss. If we do not cut the bond with the dead, they will take us with them. So, the Chinese approach is to grieve properly, and then to let go.

Part of the meaning of the Chinese character for sadness, "bei", involves a refusal of something. In this case it is a refusal to accept something sad. This sets up an inner split in the person, between reality and their psychological state. If this lasts too long, it can wear one down, and exhaust vitality. The Yellow Emperor says, "In the state of sadness and affliction one is moved at the centre, there is a drying up and life is lost" (chapter 8) (see footnote 3, p.17).

It is normal and natural to refuse to accept something sad at first, and this only becomes pathological when extended too long. In ancient China, it was said that a son should refuse to believe his father is dead for three days, but then had to accept the fact and put the body in a coffin. After that, he must cry out in affliction, and make bodily expressions of pain, when the bearers carry out the coffin.

This ritual was designed to help people come to terms with their feelings, and accept them. In fact, the bodily movements were sometimes designed to allow the qi to move properly, to counteract the qi stagnation caused by grief (see Larre p.126).

In the absence of proper grieving and mourning, pathologies can arise. The qi will stagnate in the metal organ, the lungs, and in the breast area generally, where the lung meridian flows. I have seen a number of cases of lung and breast cancer following on from bereavements which had not been dealt with.

This blockage of qi can spread to the heart too, causing it to "tighten" and to overheat. Because the heart is responsible for blood circulation, eventually there may be blood stagnation too.

Finally, this feeling of sadness can become regret. In this state, there is a kind of closure. The heart becomes "locked", and the person suffers great torment. This condition is extremely hard to treat, and one should always attempt to treat grief as early as possible.

CONFUCIUS

Confucius was born in 551 BC in the feudal state of Lu. He was recognised as a great teacher from an early age, opening his own school aged only 22. He was appointed Minister of Justice, but when the Marquis of Lu became corrupt, Confucius resigned his post, at great personal cost. He wandered about for 13 years in poverty with his disciples, seeking another state which would put his principles into practice. During this time he was often in great danger, more than once coming close to being killed, in what were very lawless times. Unable to find another state which would put his ideals into practice, he returned to his home state, and spent his last five years teaching those who would listen. He died in 478, aged 74. It was not until centuries after his death that his ideas were finally implemented as the official state philosophy of China, when the "warring states" were united in the third century BC under the Han Dynasty.

Confucius was a kind man, who inspired great loyalty in his disciples. He put his personal welfare below his high ideals, and endured great hardship for what he believed in. He was something of an ascetic, and cared little for personal comforts, although he loved music, and strongly believed in a good education to cultivate wisdom. He was known as one "who in the eager pursuit of *knowledge*, forgot his food, and in the *joy* of attaining to it forgot his sorrow" (Analects, VII, 18, see Waley 1989).

It is generally accepted that Confucius spoke more of ethics and philosophy than religion. Nevertheless, he did adhere to the traditional Chinese belief in spirits, governed at the top by the "Lord of Heaven", known as "T'ien" or "Shang di".[12] He believed in a kind of Divine Providence, and in the "Will of Heaven", which was essentially good. He taught that rulers needed the "mandate of Heaven" to rule: if they followed the will of Heaven, and were virtuous, their dynasty would thrive. If, on the other hand, rulers became corrupt, their dynasty would fall.

These ideas had a tremendous impact on the Chinese understanding of health and illness. As it was for countries (the macrocosm), so it was for the person (the microcosm). As a ruler needed to cultivate virtue in order to bring harmony to the state, so the individual needed to cultivate virtue in order to bring harmony to his body and mind. If one strays from the path of virtue, one will lose harmony, and become ill. Departure from

---

12   These two terms are still used by Chinese Christians as the name for the Christian God.

the "Will of Heaven" will bring disharmony to the person, just as it will bring disaster to the state.

With a serious illness such as cancer, there is sometimes a tendency to become self-obsessed, even self-centred. This is understandable, and to a certain degree necessary, as one searches for the way through cancer. However, what Confucius teaches us is that this must be balanced with concern for others, and for the Divine. Rather than allowing oneself to be consumed by cancer, one can strive to cultivate virtue in relation to other people, and to cultivate one's relationship to the Divine. This prevents inwardness, and a narrowing of perspective, and instead promotes an outward, upward movement. It leads towards fullness and connectedness, rather than towards emptiness and isolation. This helps one to keep a fresh perspective, and prevents one's illness from over-dominating one's life.

In order to find harmony and peace, Confucius advised the cultivation of the "Four Virtues". These have been translated in various ways, but we shall use the words sincerity, benevolence, filial piety, and propriety. Perhaps it is a mark of our times that all of these terms seem very old-fashioned. We shall look at each virtue in turn.

SINCERITY involved faithfulness, honesty, loyalty and truthfulness. It included a sense of conscientiousness and duty. It also implied a certain affection, which Confucius showed to his disciples, and which they returned. With an illness such as cancer, one has no time to waste on *in*sincerity. Through sincerity, one builds loving, trusting relationships with those around. Genuine, sincere relationships can evolve, rather than ones where the carer simply pities the person with cancer, which is all too often the case.

BENEVOLENCE was a basic attitude of generosity, and of putting the welfare of others above one's own. This virtue was thought to be rooted in man's psychology, unlike the modern view of the "selfish gene". Through helping others, one is taken out of oneself, and one's own suffering is relieved. I have seen many remarkable people with cancer devote themselves to raising money to help others with the disease, and it brought them much joy.

FILIAL PIETY consisted of love and duty towards one's parents. One can still see this virtue in operation in China, where old people are still greatly respected. Through practice of this virtue, one gains humility, which is a great virtue in itself. The respect showed to one's parents becomes a general respect for others, and helps to build a society of mutual toleration. It teaches us that we are not at the centre of all things.

PROPRIETY. The fourth virtue was propriety, which consisted of certain codes of conduct, as well as rites and rituals. Recovering a sense of ritual can be very helpful for some people with cancer, and their friends and relatives. Ritual helps one find a place of security, and helps one connect with others. Propriety also implies a sense of structure and orderliness in one's daily life, rather than chaos. When there is order, the body works more harmoniously, and the mind is calm. When there is chaos, the qi stagnates and the mind is unsettled.

Propriety also involves cultivating our relationships with the "Lord of Heaven". Without such relationships, we are incomplete and isolated. Within such relationships, we find inner peace and harmony, which has a profound impact on our state of health.

LAO TSU

Lao Tsu was an older contemporary of Confucius, and keeper of the imperial archives in the sixth century BC. According to legend he became sick at heart at the ways of men, and rode out of the city on his ox. As he was leaving, the gatekeeper persuaded him to write down his thoughts, and the result is the text the *Tao Te Ching*. In reality, however, the text was probably written for rulers, to advise them to rule according to the principles of Tao. It may well be a compilation of sayings by several people. Nevertheless, this small book, only 5000 words, has been one of the biggest influences on Chinese philosophy. It has had a deep influence on the theory and practice of Chinese medicine.

At the heart of the *Tao Te Ching* is the idea that "The universe is sacred. You cannot improve it" (v.29). The universe runs according to a certain order, a certain pattern. It runs in a certain *way*, and this way is called Tao. Likewise, man is part of this sacred cosmic order, and works in a certain *way*. If we respect this way, and live in harmony with it, we will stay healthy. If we do not live according to this way, we will become ill. Thus, the task of Chinese medicine is to return people to the way, to the Tao. This is why a key part of treatment involves educating people about how to live in tune with the sacred laws of the universe. It is no good just fixing people up so they can carry on as before. One must discover the origins of disharmony, the root of illness. When one discovers Tao, one can remain healthy: "the sage has no place for death to enter" (v.50).

Part of what Lao Tsu was referring to is what we would now call "sustainable lifestyles". It is now becoming clear that the lifestyles currently being lived by the West, and rapidly adopted by the rest of the world, are not sustainable in the long term. We are living beyond our means, both mentally, and in terms of the earth's resources. If Lao Tsu thought the society of his day had lost touch with the Tao, what would he have made of our world?

Many of the causes of cancer in the modern world are connected with our unsustainable lifestyles. We are using huge amounts of chemicals to grow our food, many of which are thought to be carcinogenic. We are experimenting with genetically modified food, despite not knowing the long-term impact this may have on both our personal health and on the wider ecosystem. We use huge amounts of cosmetics, pharmaceuticals, vaccinations, without knowing their long-term effects. It is no coincidence that as countries "develop", their rates of many kinds of cancers are soaring.

One modern, unsustainable obsession which Lao Tsu would have disapproved of is travel. He was a firm believer that wisdom is obtained by the *inner* journey, not the *outer* one, which is usually just a distraction:

> Without going outside, you may know the whole world.
> Without looking through the window, you may see the ways of heaven.
> The farther you go, the less you know.
> Thus the sage knows without travelling;
> He sees without looking. (v.47)

Indeed, it is desire for outer things that is at the root of most of our problems, and leads us into great mental confusion. To keep our minds pure and close to the Tao we would do well to avoid and ignore the advertising industry: "Not seeing desirable things prevents confusion of the heart" (v.3)… "There is no greater sin than desire, no greater curse than discontentment" (v.46). If we can let go of desire, we will find peace: "without desire there is tranquillity" (v.37). If we can only see what immeasurable gifts we have already been given by the Tao: "he who knows he has enough is rich" (v.33).

As we have seen in this book, mental confusion and a lack of tranquillity have physical effects. When the mind is disturbed, the qi does not flow properly, and becomes stagnant. Then the blood stagnates, and phlegm and toxins build up. We have seen the many treatments Chinese medicine has to offer these conditions, but if we really want to go to the root of the problem we must cultivate inner tranquillity.

Part of the Tao, according to Lao Tsu, consists in following a moral way of living (we will see later that Chuang Tsu was perhaps more ambiguous on this point). We are advised that:

> In dealing with others, be gentle and kind.
> In speech, be true.
> In ruling, be just. (v.8)

To attain Tao, we must also put others before ourselves: "through selfless action, he [the sage] attains fulfilment" (v.7). To follow our own desires at the expense of others causes a kind of closing off, a kind of narrowing. This will affect the movement of qi in a negative way. Thus, a virtuous life is a healthy life, and must be cultivated. When virtue is cultivated, it will spread outwards:

> Cultivate virtue in yourself,
> And virtue will be real.
> Cultivate it in the family,
> And virtue will abound.
> Cultivate it in the village,
> And virtue will grow.
> Cultivate it in the nation,
> And it will be abundant.
> Cultivate it in the universe,
> And it will be everywhere. (v.54)

Virtue will bring health and harmony:

> He who is filled with virtue is like a newborn child.
> Wasps and serpents will not sting him;
> Wild beasts will not pounce on him;

He will not be attacked by birds of prey...
His manhood is strong.
He screams all day without becoming hoarse.
This is perfect harmony. (v.55)

Lao Tsu tells us that we must slow down in order to find Tao. We have seen throughout this book that the fast pace of modern life causes many illnesses. It causes us to overheat, and to deplete our energy reserves. Lao Tsu said, "always be busy, and life is beyond hope" (v.52). He advises us to slow down, before we expire:

It is not wise to rush about.
Controlling the breath causes strain.
If too much energy is used, exhaustion follows.
This is not the way of Tao.
Whatever is contrary to Tao will not last long. (v.55)

On the other hand, if we slow down, we may find the Tao, the "mother of all things". This counteracts the fear which contributes to many pathologies:

Knowing the mother, one also knows the sons.
Knowing the sons, yet remaining in touch with the mother,
Brings freedom from the fear of death. (v.52)

Perhaps one of the hardest lessons Lao Tsu has for those who are very ill is to "accept misfortune and disgrace" (v.13). Most people would accept that cancer is a great misfortune. Some would also see it as a disgrace, although we argue strongly against that understanding. In any case, it is a very hard thing to accept that one has cancer. However, non-acceptance blocks the flow of qi, and can worsen illness.

Lao Tsu has had a profound influence on Chinese medicine. He advises us to slow down, to curb our desires, and to cultivate virtue. This will help our qi flow, bring mental harmony, and enhance our physical health.

CHUANG TSU

This text, known as *Wanderings on the Way*, was compiled between about the fourth and second centuries BC. The "inner chapters" were possibly written by Chuang Tsu himself, but the "outer chapters" were compiled by his followers. Unlike Confucius and Lao Tsu, Chuang Tsu does not really offer a philosophy as such. Instead, he makes fun of other philosophies, and points to the holes in them. Comparisons have been drawn between him and Socrates, for saying that it is not possible to construct any meaningful, consistent philosophy. Of course, there is an essential self-contradiction here, because this view point is itself a kind of philosophy. However, what one can certainly learn from Chuang Tsu is not to take one's model of "reality" too seriously. We can never grasp the truth in its fullness, we can only form limited approximations of it.

Whereas Lao Tsu and Confucius were making suggestions about how to improve society, Chuang Tsu concentrates more on the individual's journey. He makes no suggestions about how to improve the world, arguing that attempts to do so are usually counter productive. He argues rather that we should return to the simplicity of the "unhewn log" and the "untrained horse".

Although Chuang Tsu criticises other philosophies, he draws much from them too. We saw that Lao Tsu advised us that the Tao was sacred, so we should not try and improve it. Chuang Tsu takes up this theme with great humour:

> The emperor of the Southern Sea was Lickety, the emperor of the Northern Sea was Split, and the emperor of the centre was

Wonton. Lickety and Split often met each other in the land of Wonton, and Wonton treated them very well. Wanting to repay Wanton's kindness, Lickety and Split said "All the people have holes for seeing, hearing, eating and breathing. Wonton alone lacks them. Let's try boring some holes for him". So every day they bored one hole, and on the seventh day Wonton died. (chapter 7.7)

This story plays on a Chinese creation myth, and is saying that we should not meddle with creation. Everything has its own nature, everything manifests Tao in a different way. Man thinks he can impose a kind of structure on this, according to his own mistaken conceptions of what is best: "although a duck's legs are short, if we extend them it will come to grief; although a crane's legs are long, if we cut them short, it will be tragic".

Unlike Confucius, Chuang Tsu was wary of ritual, arguing that it stifles the true nature of things:

When Old Longears died, Idle Intruder went to mourn over him. He wailed three times and left.

"Weren't you a friend of the Master?" a disciple asked him.

"Yes."

"Well, is it proper to mourn like this?" [One would have expected a much more elaborate mourning from a friend of the dead.]

"Yes... Among those whom he had brought together, surely there were some who wished not to speak but spoke anyway, who wished not to cry but cried anyway. This is to flee from nature while redoubling human emotion, thus forgetting what we have received from nature. This was what the ancients called "the punishment for fleeing from nature"... One who is situated in timeliness and who dwells in favourableness can not be affected by joy or sorrow. This is what the ancients called the emancipation of the gods." (chapter 3.5)

Instead of following ritual expression, Chuang Tsu encouraged the spontaneous expression of emotion. To regulate such matters was to go against Tao. Every person will feel things in a different way, and should be left to find their own personal expression of Tao. There is no one correct size for all, and Tao will be expressed differently by each person.

In terms of Chinese medicine, Chuang Tsu's philosophy of spontaneity and creativity can be linked with the wood element. Free flow of ideas and emotions leads to free flow of liver qi (governed by wood). If we are overly constricted by rules, preconceptions, and logic our qi flow may be inhibited. We can look for a balance between Chuang Tsu's freedom, and the firmer guidelines suggested by Confucius. Chuang Tsu would certainly not have approved of the kind of "freedom" we crave in our society. It would strike him as very self-centred, and very grasping. In fact his "freedom" required much struggle to attain, unlike the easy freedom of our society.

Chuang Tsu offers a great lesson on illness and suffering:

Sir Chariot fell ill. When Sir Sacrifice went to call on him, Sir Chariot said, "Great is the Creator of all things! She's making me all crookedy like this!" His back was all hunched up. On top were his five dorsal introductories. His chin was buried in his bellybutton. His shoulders were higher than the crown of his head. His neck bones were pointing to the sky. His vital yin yang breaths were out of kilter. Yet his mind was at ease, as though nothing were amiss. He hobbled over to a well and looked at his reflection in the water. "Alas" he said. "The Creator of Things is making me all crookedy like this!"

"Do you resent it?" asked Sir Sacrifice.

"No. Why should I resent it? Supposing my left arm were transformed into a chicken, I would consequently go looking for a rooster that could call out the hours of the night. Supposing that my right arm were transformed into a crossbow, I would consequently go looking for an owl to roast. Supposing that my buttocks were transformed into wheels and my spirit into a horse, I would consequently mount upon them. What need would I for any other conveyance? Furthermore, what we attain is due to timeliness, and what we lose is the result of compliance. If we repose in timeliness and dwell in compliance, sorrow and joy cannot affect us. This is what the ancients called "emancipation". (chapter 6.5)

However bad things get, there is always room for humour. Whatever mess one is in, one can always find something positive to say. If we learn to accept whatever we attain, and whatever we lose, we are free of worry.

We can also learn from this quote that one can suffer from cancer, while displaying great maturity of spirit. Although in Chinese medicine physical weakness can lead to weakness of spirit, a very strong spirit can overcome physical and emotional problems. "Princely Nag" had been mutilated by having a foot cut off, but saw this loss merely as the "sloughing off of a clump of earth".

Chuang Tsu did not set out to offer a coherent philosophy. He is open to criticisms of harking back to a non-existent ideal past, and advocating anarchy. Nevertheless, we can learn much about health and wholeness from him. He reminds us not to take ourselves too seriously, and to cultivate a child-like simplicity and playfulness. He teaches us not to ever think we have all the answers. He teaches us to accept whatever comes our way, and to love this great gift of life, despite the suffering it involves.

MONOTHEISM

The worship of a personal God played a central part in Chinese culture for over 4000 years, and any discussion of self-cultivation would be incomplete without some understanding of this. From at least 2205 BC Chinese emperors offered an annual sacrifice to Shang Di, which can be translated as "Most High God" or "Lord Above". This ritual came to be known as the "Border Sacrifice", and continued until 1911, when the Manchu dynasty was overthrown. It involved the sacrifice of a young, unblemished bull on an outdoor altar, by the emperor, who acted as high priest. In the 15th century AD, the ceremony was transferred to the huge and magnificent Temple of Heaven complex, which is still in existence in Beijing.

The ceremony was a vast and colourful event, involving large numbers of people, dressed in colourful silk clothes, and playing bells, drums, cymbals, flutes and stringed instruments, dedicated solely for the event. The emperor would pray:

> To Thee, O mysteriously working maker, I look up in thought… With the great ceremonies I reverently honour Thee. Thy servant, I am but a reed or willow; my heart is but that of an ant; yet I have received thy favouring decree, appointing me to the government of the empire… Come in Thy precious chariot to the altar. Thy servant, I bow my head to the earth reverently, expecting Thine abundant grace… All human beings, all things of the earth, rejoice together in His Great Name.[13]

Shang Di was conceived as the creator of all: "When Di had so decreed, He called into existence heaven, earth, and man.

---

13 Original translation by James Legge, in "The Notions of the Chinese Concerning God and Spirits" (Hong Kong: Hong Kong Register Office, 1852), p.52. Reproduced in Nelson, Broadberry & Chock (1997) *God's promise to the Chinese*, Read Books, p.4–5.

Between heaven and earth He separately placed in order men and things, all overspread by the heavens".[14]

There are many striking parallels between Shang Di and the God of the Hebrews, not least in the name: the Jewish name for God which was in use around 2000 BC was "El Shaddai", very similar to Shang Di. China's earliest writings, inscribed in about 1500 BC on tortoise shells, appear to tell of events similar to those narrated in Genesis. They appear to show God shaping man from the earth, and making him holy, in the image of God. The man appears to be placed in a garden with four rivers, similar to Eden. A woman is created for the man, and then the two fall away from God in disobedience. The geographical origins of Genesis were not so far from China (in what is now Iraq), and it has been speculated that the events narrated in Genesis, and the knowledge of the Creator God, also found their way east into China.

For Confucius, an understanding of the worship of Shang Di was crucial to self-cultivation: "He who understands the ceremonies of the sacrifices to Heaven and Earth...would find the government of a kingdom as easy as to look into his palm".[15] For Confucius, a correct relationship with God was the basis for a correct relationship with other people. This relationship was maintained by the sacrificial ritual, which set the tone of how one should relate to God. This is one of the reasons why ritual was one of the Confucian virtues (as we saw above). But we must also bear in mind that ritual was not enough in itself: without a corresponding inner movement of the heart, ritual would be devoid of its true meaning and purpose.

It could be argued that as Taoism became more popular, focus on the *personal* God, Shang Di, was often replaced by a

---

14   ibid, p.20.
15   ibid, p.2.

focus on a more *impersonal* "Tao". In addition, one could also argue that the border ceremony became somewhat corrupted, by focusing more on the person of the emperor than on Shang Di Himself. Nevertheless, Shang Di continued to play an important role in China for four millennia, and this is often reflected in Chinese medical thought. For example, just as the emperor mediated between God and man within the *empire*, the heart mediated between God and man in the *individual*. The heart is the organ which houses the shen, or spirit, through which we relate to the Divine.

SUMMARY

In this chapter we have looked at some of the philosophical ideas that shaped Chinese medicine. We have seen that development of the mind is generally reflected in a healthy body. We have also seen that if the mind is cultivated to a high degree, bodily afflictions and suffering can be born much more readily.

The various philosophers each have different lessons for us. Some emphasised the importance of cultivating virtue, and following the "Way of Heaven", as governed by a personal "Lord of Heaven". Others talked of striving towards a less personal "Tao", which involves a more natural lifestyle. Some strived to create a better *society,* while others emphasised the *personal* quest for wisdom. Some emphasised the need for struggle, while others emphasised the need for a more playful, humorous approach.

All, however, agreed that the cultivation of one's spirit is a key part of maintaining health, wholeness and harmony.

FURTHER READING

Damascene, H. (2002) *Christ The Eternal Tao.* Platina, CA: Valaam Press.

English, J. and Gia Fu Feng (trans) (1972) *Lao Tsu – The Tao Te Ching.* Farnham, UK: Gower.

Larre, C. (1996) *The Seven Emotions.* Cambridge, UK: Monkey Press.

Mair, V. (1994) *Wandering on the Way – Early Taoist Tales and Parables of Chuang Tsu.* New York, NY: Bantam Books.

Maoshing, Ni. (trans) (1995) *The Yellow Emperor's Classic of Internal Medicine.* Boston, MA: Shambhala.

Merton, T. (1965) *The Way of Chuang Tsu.* New York, NY: New Directions.

Nelson, E. R., Broadberry, R. E. and Chock, G. T. (1997) *Gods Promise to the Chinese.* Dunlap, TN: Read Books.

Waley, A. (1989) *The Analects of Confucius.* New York, NY: Vintage.

CHAPTER THREE

Celestial Lancets: Acupuncture in the Management of Cancer

CHAPTER CONTENTS

WHAT IS ACUPUNCTURE?

Acupuncture is the insertion of fine needles into the skin. The needles are much finer than hypodermic needles, as they do not have fluids passing through them. The patient will feel little or no pain on insertion. Once the needle is inserted, the practitioner will turn the needle slightly until the patient feels a sensation around the needle. Patients describe this sensation in various ways, such as heat, tingling, numbness, electricity, heaviness, or a dull ache. Some patients will feel sensations in a different part of the body to where the needle was inserted, most commonly along the course of the acupuncture channel that has been needled. This sensation indicates the "arrival of qi" at the point, what the Chinese call "de qi".

The number of needles used in one session is usually between about six to 12. The needles are usually retained for about 15 to 20 minutes, although in some styles they may be removed as soon as the qi arrives. Single use, disposable needles should be used. Usually patients require a course of treatments to get the full benefits of acupuncture. Acupuncture has a cumulative effect, a bit like exercise: one has to do a certain amount in order to make progress. Acupuncture attempts to re-pattern the flow of qi in the body, to break the body's old habitual patterns, which takes time. Some patients' qi responds very quickly to acupuncture, while others' qi takes longer. We have a rough rule of thumb for acupuncture that for every year of imbalance, one month of treatment is required.

Acupuncture aims to restore the free flow of qi in the meridian system. As we have seen, a major cause of illness, especially cancer, is stagnation of qi. Through detailed diagnosis, the practitioner will establish exactly where the qi is blocked, and attempt to move it with acupuncture. We shall look in more detail below at the meridian system, which is highly complex, and takes many years for practitioners to grasp in its fullness.

With western medical research, the personality of the therapist is deliberately excluded from clinical trials: the quality and attitude of the doctor should not influence the outcome. Conversely, for acupuncturists it is recognised that qualities such as empathy have a huge impact on the healing process. The acupuncturist is trained to work from the heart, and to cultivate a good relationship with the patient. It is recognised that the quality of energy in the practitioner profoundly influences the quality of energy in the patient. If the practitioner is calm and centred, then the patient will absorb some of this. Conversely, if the practitioner is nervous, the patient may become nervous.

The switch

During acupuncture, most people find that they become very relaxed (as noted, this depends to a certain degree on the practitioner). Many patients say that they are able to "let go" of problems in their lives during a session, and for some time afterwards. One explanation for this is that acupuncture helps the patient's nervous system to switch from the *sympathetic* state to the *parasympathetic* state. When one is in the sympathetic state, one is ready for "fight or flight", in other words ready for action. It is appropriate to be in this state when one has to go to work, or do other active things. In this state, the blood flows to the muscles and brain in readiness for action.

The other branch of the nervous system is the parasympathetic state. When one has finished work, and it is time to rest, one needs to switch into this state, where the blood supply flows to the internal organs. In this state, the body can repair itself, and the organs can do the work of digesting food and breaking down toxins.

Problems arise when people get stuck in the sympathetic state, and are unable to switch to the parasympathetic state. This happens when one is in a state of chronic stress. In this state, instead of resting from time to time, one just keeps going until one collapses. When people get stuck in this state, they are unable to repair and rebuild cells properly. They are unable to extract the nutrients from their food. They are unable to break down and excrete toxins. If one remains in this state for an extended period, months or years, one can become very ill. One will lack essential nutrients, and toxins will accumulate. Body tissue will start to become damaged, and cells will not function properly.

This pattern of being stuck in sympathetic mode, in "fight or flight state", is often one of the key contributory factors in many cancers. The problem is exacerbated by receiving a diagnosis of cancer, which will cause further stress. The conventional treatment of cancer can also increase stress levels, by causing further pain and discomfort.

This is why acupuncture can be so helpful for such people. By showing the nervous system how to switch back to the parasympathetic state, patients are enabled to relax at last. The body can start to repair itself, and the person finds a kind of "breathing space" in their lives. One patient said to me that acupuncture allowed her to stop being like a "hamster stuck on a wheel". It allowed her to step back from her hectic life, and to see it more objectively. Rather than always being caught up in the busyness of daily activity, acupuncture helped her to see the bigger picture. This helped her to plan and live her life more fully.

Initially, this relaxing effect usually lasts for a day or two. After a course of treatments the change tends to become more permanent. This is because the person's nervous system can gradually learn to switch *by itself* into the parasympathetic state. The acupuncture shows it what to do, and over time it learns to do it by itself. Acupuncture helps the nervous system to establish new patterns. The human is a creature of habit, and this reflects the tendency of our nervous system to work in certain habitual pathways. With a course of acupuncture, the nervous system can establish new, more helpful habits.

Often people don't realise that they are exhausted. I asked one patient how her energy level was, and she replied "fine". I asked her how her energy level would be if she stopped drinking coffee. After a pause she replied, "I would probably not be able to function". Many people keep themselves stimulated by coffee, cigarettes, sugary foods, drugs, loud music or "excitement". When such people receive acupuncture, they can leave the treatment room feeling very tired. Acupuncture switches off the production of adrenaline that has kept them going, so they actually feel how tired their bodies really are. We have forgotten the function of tiredness: to tell us to rest.

The extent to which acupuncture can bring positive changes depends greatly on the patient. People who are willing to examine their patterns of thought and behaviour tend to respond much better than those who aren't. Whereas western medicine tries to force the body to mend, Chinese medicine tries to persuade the body–mind to heal. The co-operation of the patient is required. We examined what patients can do to facilitate their acupuncture in the chapter on cultivating the spirit. The acupuncture is offering to teach us something, it is up to us how carefully we listen. As Confucius said: "I hold up one quarter of the lesson to my pupils, it is up to them to return with the other three quarters."

Acupuncture points and the structure of the universe

I am often asked whether acupuncture points have any basis in physical reality. While we cannot fully explain how they work, modern research has shed some light on them. Acupuncture points are small areas of high electrical conductivity (or, put another way, areas of low electrical resistance). With appropriate equipment, the level of conductivity can be measured to be higher than that of the surrounding skin. When a person is ill in a particular organ, the level of conductivity tends to rise to an even higher level in acupoints associated with that organ. When acupuncture is administered to the relevant points, the level of conductivity tends to fall back towards the normal level. We can therefore say that acupuncture is associated with the electrical systems of the body, with "bioelectricity". We also know that cellular activity is profoundly influenced by electrical fields, so we can hypothesise that acupuncture may work by changing electrical fields in the body.

It has also been shown that the insertion of acupuncture needles causes immediate changes in the electrical activity of the brain. Insertion into a point called Large Intestine 4 causes pain control centres in the brain to become active. In one experiment, insertion of needles into patients with Alzheimer's disease activated brain centres associated with cognitive functions.[16]

A medical physicist in the United States, Cho Zang-Hee, who pioneered the proton emission tomography (PET) scanner, became interested in acupuncture when it helped his back injury. Cho had an acupuncturist needle various people in an acupoint at the side of the little toe (the bladder meridian), which is connected with the eyes. In one person after another, the visual cortex lit up, just as if they had been stimulated with a flash of light. Inserting the needle into a non-acupoint in the big toe had no effect.[17]

Physicist Mae Wan Ho, Director of the Institute of Science in Society, has recently made remarkable discoveries about the energy structures in living organisms. She has developed revolutionary optical imaging techniques, which demonstrate that organisms are so "dynamically coherent" at the molecular level that they *appear* to have liquid crystalline structures. These structures exist in every cell in the body, and allow for instant, non-local, communication within the whole body. This communication may occur via "proton jump-conduction". This "is telling us that the living organism is coherent beyond our wildest dreams, with dynamic order that extends from the molecular to the macroscopic".[18] Ho goes on:

---

16   As measured by a functional magnetic resonance imaging machine. See *Acupuncture and Electro-therapeutics Research* 2008;33(1–2);9–17.

17   Dr. Mae-Wan Ho: "Coherent Energy, Liquid Crystallinity and Acupuncture", talk given to the British Acupuncture Society, 2 October, 1999.

18   Ibid.

Liquid crystallinity gives organisms their characteristic flexibility, exquisite sensitivity and responsiveness, thus optimizing the rapid, noiseless intercommunication that enables the organism to function as a coherent, coordinated whole. In addition, the liquid crystalline continuum provides subtle electrical interconnections which are sensitive to changes in pressure, pH and other physicochemical conditions; in other words, it is also able to register "tissue memory". Thus, the liquid crystalline continuum possesses all the qualities of a "body consciousness" that may indeed be sensitive to all forms of subtle energy medicines including acupuncture.

Ho thinks that collagen, which is connective tissue found throughout the human body, may be the main medium by which communication occurs. The electrical properties of collagen make it very responsive to tiny changes in electrical signals. She says: "Aligned collagen fibres in connective tissues provide oriented channels for electrical intercommunication, and are strongly reminiscent of acupuncture meridians in traditional Chinese medicine."

According to Ho's model, consciousness is not localised in the brain, but penetrates the whole being. The whole body is a unified, "conscious" structure, with internal coherence. This accords very well with the Chinese notion that the qi system stores emotions and consciousness, and that acupuncture can therefore access them. She concludes that:

Western medicine, by contrast [to Chinese medicine], has yet no concept of the whole, and is based, at the very outset, on a Cartesian divide between mind and brain, and brain and body. Because there is no concept of the organism as a whole, there is, in effect, no theory of health, only an infinite number of disease models, each based on the supposed defect of a single molecular species. There is an urgent need to develop a theory of health for proper delivery of healthcare in the next millennium.

The implications for our understanding of cancer are enormous. We can no longer think of it as a *local* problem: it is an imbalance of the *whole* organism. Local cellular malfunctions can not be seen in isolation from the rest of the person, but rather reflect a distortion of the whole organism. Treatment must therefore address the whole organism.

One could speculate that the kind of fields described by Ho extend in some way *outside* of the physical body, in the same way as the Chinese think of the human qi system as embedded in larger energy fields. *Acupuncture points could be the interface between our own personal internal energy systems and the wider systems around us.* In other words, they are not just treating the person, they are modulating her relationship with the outside world.

At the ultimate level there could be a kind of universal matrix within which all organisms exist. According to this kind of model, we are no longer isolated entities, but are all connected together in the web of life. There is a dynamic exchange between our own personal energy fields which affects the wider fields around us.

This takes us away from the "Newtonian" system of isolated units, randomly colliding from time to time, like billiard balls. It moves us towards a perception of the universe as structured and integrated. For me, this suggests that the universe is filled with meaning and purpose, and the work of a Creator: how could something so beautifully coherent have occurred by chance, without any design? I'm well aware that many others will not draw this conclusion, but I think it is at least fair to say that acupuncture and the "new physics" are by no means inconsistent with the idea of God.

It has been said of western medicine that it is about one hundred years behind physics. Chinese medicine, on the other hand, seems to fit very well with the "new physics".

A HISTORY OF ACUPUNCTURE

The earliest historical references to acupuncture date from the sixth century BC. One such reference is the Tso Chuan commentary on the Chhun Chhiu, a record of the affairs of the feudal states between the eight and fifth centuries BC. The Prince of Chin is gravely ill, and so the Prince of Chhin sends his Doctor Huan to attend him:

> Having arrived...the physician (Huan) said: "This disease is incurable. It has settled in the region between the heart and the diaphragm... No needle can penetrate to it, no drug can reach it. There is nothing to be done." The Prince exclaimed, "what an excellent physician!" Then he caused him to be treated with honour, and sent him back to Chhin.[19]

Needham comments that:

> Perhaps not every patient nowadays would applaud so selflessly the honesty of his doctor, though some may appreciate more candour than they actually get; in any case the story is another indication of the very rational and scientific spirit which animated the early centuries of Chinese medicine.

At this time, it seems that needles were made of stone, bamboo and bone: bone needles still survive from the Neolithic period. They would obviously not have been fine enough to perform acupuncture as we now know it, and would probably have been

---

19   Quoted in Needham, J. *et al.* (2002) *Celestial Lancets: A History and Rationale of Acupuncture and Moxa.* London: Routledge, p.78.

used for a kind of blood letting, whereby "evil influences" were purged from the body. As metalworking developed, metal needles were made, and specimens of bronze needles from the third century BC still exist. By the second century BC, there was a well established steel industry in China, producing steel needles. With the advent of this technology, the art of acupuncture was enabled to flourish. Crude methods of bloodletting were gradually replaced by subtle methods of manipulating the qi.

Indeed, it is from the second century onwards that we see increasingly complex charts showing the locations of acupuncture points. By the time of the Yellow Emperor (around second to first century BC), the art of acupuncture had become fairly complex, as the following quotation shows:

> Huang Ti [the Yellow Emperor] said: "I should like to know the Tao of acupuncture." Qi Bo replied: "The first thing in this art and mystery is that you must concentrate the mind...then, once you have decided on the state of his five viscera (whether deficient or excess), as indicated by the nine pulse observations, you can take the needle in hand. If you have felt no deathlike pulse, and heard no inauspicious sound, then the inner and outer signs are in correspondence. You must not rely on the external appearances (symptoms) only, and you must understand fully the coming and going of the qi in the meridians; then alone can you perform acupuncture on the patient."[20]

The Yellow Emperor gives detailed anatomical descriptions of the main acupuncture meridians, and discusses diseases related to each meridian. This knowledge was developed and disseminated, and by the second century AD acupuncture was in universal use throughout China.[21]

---

20 Quoted in Needham *et al.* p.91. Note: grammar altered to improve style, and Pin Yin used for consistency with the rest of this book. (See Footnote 19.)

21 Needham *et al.* p.118. (See Footnote 19.)

In the 11th century, life-size bronze figures were cast, with small holes for each of the acupuncture points. The figures were covered with wax to hide the holes, and filled with water. As part of their examinations, students had to needle the points correctly, allowing water to come out of the holes. Failure to produce the water would mean the student had failed his exam. When my acupuncture students complain about how hard their exams are, I tell them about the bronze figures.

By this time, the number of recognised acupuncture points had stabilised at around 350 (some texts listed an idealised 365 points, to correspond with the number of days in the year). This is still the number of main points recognised today.

The theoretical basis of acupuncture has continued to evolve to the current day. However, it is interesting that most of the basic theories underlying acupuncture have changed little in two thousand years.

THE MERIDIAN SYSTEM

The human microcosm

We saw in Chapter One that qi flows in channels, called meridians. There are 12 ordinary meridians, and eight "extra-ordinary meridians". Each of the 12 ordinary meridians is connected to an organ. Each ordinary meridian starts at the tip either of a finger or a toe. Six of the 12 start in a finger, and six start in a toe. The meridians run along the limb, and then into the torso, to join with their organ. As well as the main branch of the meridian, there are numerous smaller branches, connecting the meridians to each other.

The meridians are the same on both sides of the body. In other words, each side is a mirror of the other.

We can compare the meridians to a map of the London Underground train system. Each of the 12 main meridians could be thought of as a certain line: the lungs could be the Piccadilly Line, and the kidneys could be the Northern Line, for example. The lines all connect up at various points, so one can travel seamlessly anywhere on the system. However, if there are engineering works causing a delay somewhere, problems will be caused throughout the system.

Again, we can see the *interconnectedness* of Chinese medicine: a problem in one area will soon spread to others, and eventually the whole system will grind to a halt. When the transport system breaks down, substances are not moved around properly, so blockages and deficiencies will arise. Confusion, delay, and general irritability will result.

Along the meridians, there are located acupuncture points, or acupoints for short. We can think of these acupoints as stations on our underground network. At these stations, people can enter or exit the underground system. At these points, qi can enter or exit the body. If the patient has an *excess* of qi in a certain place, acupuncture can get rid of that excess. If the patient has a *deficiency* of qi, acupuncture can hep to gather more qi. The acupuncturist has different techniques which are used either to disperse or gather the qi.

The analogy of an underground train system is similar to the ancient Chinese analogy of an irrigation system for the meridian network. Indeed, many names of acupoints are taken from irrigation systems. If the system is working properly, all the crops will receive just the right amount of water. If there are any blockages, the crops will die from drought or flood.

According to some ancient Chinese doctors, each meridian was a microcosm of a certain constellation, and the meridian system as a whole was seen as a microcosm of the whole cosmos, a personification of the whole universe. Imbalance in the human would lead to imbalance in whole cosmos. It is interesting to note the parallel here with the Christian teaching that when Adam (mankind) fell from grace, the whole cosmos went out of kilter. Such ideas are at the root of the Confucian notion that one must cultivate virtue in oneself, in order to benefit the whole universe (which we explored further in the chapter on cultivation of the spirit).

Some key meridians and points

A good knowledge of the meridian system is fundamental to working with cancer. One of the first tasks is to identify which meridians may be involved in the development of the cancer. Only then can an attempt be made to restore the proper flow of qi in the affected meridian. By correcting the qi imbalances which lead to the cancer developing, and by promoting qi flow into the affected area, acupuncture aims to help the body recover, and to minimise the chance of recurrence.

It takes many years to master the complexities of the meridian system. We can only give here the briefest sample of some key meridians and acupuncture points, to give a flavour of how acupuncture works.

THE KIDNEY MERIDIAN

As we saw in Chapter One, the kidneys are vital organs in Chinese medicine. They help determine the constitution and overall vitality of the person. The kidney meridian starts on the sole of the foot, and runs up the inside of the leg. It connects with two "extra-ordinary meridians" which flow into the reproductive organs. A branch runs into the lumbar spine. The meridian then runs up the front of the chest, and a branch goes into the throat and tongue.

As with all the meridians, if there is an imbalance in the organ system, this may cause problems along the course of the meridian. Thus, kidney problems may be associated with cancers of the reproductive system (such as uterine, ovarian and prostate), and spinal cancers. They may also contribute to the development of cancer of the throat.

The first point on the kidney channel, on the sole of the foot, is called "Gushing Spring". The name can be interpreted in a number of ways. When the point is needled, patients sometimes have the sensation that a jet of water is gushing into the point. Also, the kidney is governed by the element water, so the point is used to nourish the water of the body. Just as water is the source of life and vitality, so "Gushing Spring" provides life and vitality to the body.

The next point on the kidney meridian, Kidney 2, is called "Blazing Valley". The Chinese character for yin is a valley, so this point is used to treat hot flushes caused by kidney yin deficiency. This point is commonly used to treat flushes due to radiotherapy, or to the drug Tamoxifen, which can cause kidney yin deficiency.

THE LIVER MERIDIAN

The liver meridian starts in the big toe, and runs up the inner leg. It wraps around the genitals, and then spreads through the chest and into the breasts. A branch runs up to the top of the head, to the point known as "One Hundred Meetings" (Bai Hui). Liver imbalances can manifest in cancers involving the genitals, especially cervical cancer. They can also manifest in breast cancer.

One of the most important points on the body is Liver 3, "Great Rushing". Liver qi stagnation contributes to many cancers, and this is one of the mot important points to unblock stuck liver qi. When needled, this point can cause the stuck qi to rush forth, hence the name of the point. On a mental level, the point can cause a release of pent up emotions, especially anger and frustration. When needled together with Large Intestine 4, the combination is known as the "Four Gates". This can be a very powerful treatment, which can open the flood gates, so the stagnant qi can rush through.

Above the ankle is a point called "Woodworm Canal" (Liver 5). This point opens a small connecting channel which runs from the liver to the gall bladder meridian. These two meridians belong to the wood element, hence the name of the point indicating a canal being burrowed through the wood. This point treats a "knot of stuck qi, like a stone", below the navel. It is therefore indicated for cancers in this area. It is also very powerful at treating some of the emotions which commonly accompany cancer, such as worry, oppression, depression, fear, and fright. It also treats the sensation of stuckness in the throat, known as "globus hystericus" by western medicine: because nothing physical can be found in the throat, the condition is dismissed as "all in the mind" (that is, the patient is hysterical!). In Chinese medicine this blockage is due to phlegm, and is treated with this point. Finally, Woodworm Canal also helps to clear the liver of heat toxins, which can play a role in cancer.

The last point on the liver meridian, Liver 14, is called "Cycle Gate", because it is the last point in the cycle of qi around the body. The qi begins its cycle at Lung 1, then runs through all 12 primary meridians, before completing the circuit at "Cycle Gate", and returning to Lung 1 to begin the cycle again. Cycle Gate is located just below the breast, and is indicated for breast cancer. The liver meridian has a powerful influence on the breast: premenstrual breast lumps are an indication of liver qi stagnation. If it is not possible to needle the side of the body where the cancer is/was, one can needle the same point on the opposite side of the body. When any point on the body is needled, it works on both sides of the body.

When the qi is stagnant in the liver channel, it can affect the stomach channel, which runs nearby. This is a pattern known as "liver attacking stomach", which prevents the qi from descending in the stomach channel, causing nausea. Needling Cycle Gate will treat this problem.

THE HEART MERIDIAN

The heart meridian starts in the armpit, and runs down the inside of the arm to the little finger. People having heart attacks feel pain radiating down the meridian.

As we have seen, the heart is the centre of the emotional life in Chinese medicine. Cancer will inevitably cause emotional upsets, and points from the heart channel are used to treat these. The most common point used is usually "Door of the Spirit", Heart 7. This point has a very calming effect, and is used for a wide range of emotional problems, such as anxiety, fear, dread, panic, shock, insomnia, and palpitations.

THE PERICARDIUM MERIDIAN

This organ is known as the "heart protector" in Chinese medicine, and its function is to protect the heart from undue stress. The heart is known as the emperor, and the pericardium as the emperor's minister. The emperor is protected from daily worries and cares by his minister, so he can concentrate on the higher matters of running the empire. Similarly, the heart is protected so it can focus on the loftier concerns of the spirit.

The point Pericardium 5 is called "Intermediary Messenger", indicating its role as a minister for the emperor. It is an important point to treat phlegm in the chest, which may cause breast cancer. Phlegm can lodge in the heart, causing mental confusion, and a feeling of being cut off from the world. We call this situation "phlegm misting the heart", and this point treats this condition well.

Pericardium 6 is known as "Inner Pass", and again, we have a sense of a secret inner route to the heart, known only to the minister. It is also known as "Inner Block", as it is very effective at freeing blockages from the chest area, and from the mind too. It is used with cancers in the chest area, such as lung and breast. One branch of the pericardium channel descends into the lower abdomen, and this point helps stuck qi to descend, thus effectively treating nausea. We will see below that there is evidence for the effectiveness of this point in treating nausea caused by chemotherapy.

THE DIGESTION ("SPLEEN") MERIDIAN

This meridian runs close to the liver, from the big toe into the chest. Its inner branches enter the intestines and stomach, and it is indicated for cancers in those areas. Many points on this channel are used to clear phlegm, and while they will not clear a tumour, they may prevent phlegm building up again and causing a recurrence.

Spleen 4 is called "Gong Sun", which is the family name of the Yellow Emperor. Chinese history is divided into phases, corresponding to the Five Elements, and the Yellow Emperor ruled in the Earth phase. The digestive system is related to the Earth element.

This point is used when the patient takes no pleasure in eating, which is a common complaint associated with chemotherapy. It is also used when food does not move properly through the intestines, and the patient feels over-full or nauseous. This point is very helpful to treat worry, the emotion associated with the digestive system.

Spleen 6 is called "Three Yin Intersection", because the three yin channels of the leg meet there, namely the liver, kidneys and digestion ("spleen"). The point therefore treats all three organs. It is particularly useful with cancer, as it clears both phlegm and stagnant blood. It also has a powerful effect on a wide range of emotions, and because it is very yin has a very calming effect. Because it treats both kidneys and spleen, organs responsible for water metabolism, it can help treat oedema, a common problem in cancer patients. Because it nourishes the yin, it is used to help generate fluids in cases of xerostomia (the inability to produce adequate saliva following radiation damage to the salivary gland). **NB: this point is used to induce labour, and is therefore contra-indicated in pregnancy.**

Spleen 10 is known as the "Sea of Blood". It has the dual action of both nourishing and invigorating blood. It is therefore commonly used in cancers due to blood stagnation.

Spleen 21 is called "Great Wrapping". This is because a network of channels runs from this point, on the side of the chest, and wraps around the whole chest area. This point has a profound effect on the breasts, and is indicated in breast and lung cancer. It is also indicated when the patient has pain throughout their whole body, combined with a sense of weariness, both physically and mentally. It is a very helpful point when patients are feeling battle weary in their struggle against cancer. This point also treats weak limbs, as the digestive system governs the limbs. It also helps with chest pain and coughing in cases of lung cancer.

THE LUNG MERIDIAN

The lung channel runs from the chest to the thumbs, and is needled in cases of lung cancer. Several lung points help to move qi and disperse phlegm throughout the whole chest. They are particularly relevant in the presence of grief, the emotion associated with the lungs.

Lung 3 is called "Palace of Heaven". It is one of the ten "Window of Heaven" points, identified in the *Yellow Emperor* text. These points often have a calming effect on the emotions, and indeed Lung 3 is used with sadness, weeping, and mental disorientation. It is also used when patients cannot sleep at night, but can not stay awake during the day.

WHAT CAN ACUPUNCTURE OFFER THOSE WITH CANCER?

Chinese medicine generally holds that acupuncture is not strong enough to get rid of cancer by itself. Acupuncture is effective in promoting the flow of qi, but if there is a build up of phlegm, blood stagnation, and heat toxins, as we have with tumours, acupuncture will probably not be sufficient to remove them. So what benefits can acupuncture provide in the management of cancer? In this section we can provide only a small selection of the benefits acupuncture can bring to those with cancer.

We must also remember that although much of the research we quote attempts to measure the treatment of single symptoms, acupuncture by its very nature treats the whole person. Even when we focus on treating symptoms, it is done within the context of the overall energetic pattern of the patient. One always treats the *root* and the *branch*, the *underlying pattern* and the *disease manifestation*.

Pain control

Pain can be caused by cancer itself, or by surgery. According to Chinese medicine, blocked qi flow will tend to increase pain levels. We say "where there is pain there is no free flow of qi; where there is free flow of qi, there is no pain". One of the benefits of acupuncture over drugs is that it will help the patient to relax, and help their qi flow. Rather than just removing the pain signal, acupuncture helps to reduce pain at its source. Painkilling drugs can also induce unpleasant side effects, such as fatigue (which is often a problem anyway). Any other techniques which have an analgesic (painkilling) effect are therefore very welcome. Acupuncture has long been used to control pain, and modern research is uncovering some of the mechanisms of how it might do so.

Many acupoints lie near peripheral nerve beds, and it has been suggested that the analgesic effect of acupuncture is mediated through these nerve beds. This hypothesis was supported by the discovery that the analgesic effect is blocked by the local administration of lidocaine (which impairs the function of the nerve beds).[22]

The analgesic effect of acupuncture may also be partly explained by Melzack and Wall's "gate theory" of pain. This theory suggests that there are "gates" in the spinal cord which only allow one kind of sensory signal through at once. If a sensory signal is given by acupuncture, it may block the pain signal.[23]

It has also been shown that the systemic (i.e. whole body) analgesic effect of acupuncture is produced by certain opioids, namely beta endorphin and met-enkephalin. Several studies have shown elevated levels of these chemicals after acupuncture. When chemicals are given which prevent these opioids working, the pain is no longer controlled by acupuncture, suggesting that it is indeed these opioids which are controlling the pain.[24]

---

22   Cohen *et al.*, *Integrative Cancer Therapies* 2005;4(2):131–43.
23   Op cit.
24   Op cit.

Since the 1990s, researchers have been able to monitor the activity of the pain control centres in the brain, using new scanning techniques such as positron emission tomography (PET) and functional magnetic resonance imaging (fMRI). In 2005 a systematic review was undertaken into the use of these techniques to monitor the effects of acupuncture on the brain's pain centres.[25] The reviewers found a number of research projects which suggested that acupuncture activated certain areas of the brain associated with pain control.

Various researchers have compared the effects of acupuncture at *traditional* acupoints with acupuncture at *non-acupoints*. It has been found that inserting a needle anywhere has an effect on some pain control centres in the brain, but inserting a needle at an acupoint has a far greater effect.[26] In any case, it is becoming clear that the physiological effects of acupuncture are extremely complex, involving many areas of the brain, and many of the body's chemicals.[27]

One study examined the use of auricular (ear) acupuncture for cancer pain. Ninety subjects were divided into three groups, the therapeutic group receiving auricular acupuncture at certain key points (these points were defined as areas of lowered electrical resistance, as discussed above).[28] The two control groups

---

25   Lewis *et al.*, *Evidence Based Complementary and Alternative Medicine* 2005 September;2(3):315–19.

26   Wu *et al.*, *Neuroimage* 2002 Aug;16(4):1028–37. NB: This study looked at electro-acupuncture, which we shall examine below.

27   One piece of research suggested that "recent evidence shows that nitric oxide plays an important role in mediating the cardiovascular responses to EA [electro-acupuncture] stimulation through the gracile nucleus-thalamic pathway. Other substances, including serotonin, catecholamines, inorganic chemicals and amino acids such as glutamate and α-aminobutyric acid (GABA), are proposed to mediate certain cardiovascular and analgesic effects of acupuncture, but at present their role is poorly understood". *Evidence Based Complementary and Alternative Medicine* 2004 June;1(1):41–47.

28   The electrical properties of these points allowed the measurement of an electro-dermal signal.

received sham auricular acupuncture at other points on the ear, where there was no electrical signal. Pain was measured two months into the trial, using a visual analog score (VAS). The study found that "pain intensity decreased by 36 per cent at two months from baseline in the group receiving acupuncture; there was little change for patients receiving placebo (2%). The difference between groups was statistically significant".[29] This study also supports the idea discussed above, that the way acupuncture controls pain is connected with the electrical properties of acupoints.

Enhanced immunity

Chronic stress can undermine many of the body's systems, and this is particularly true of the immune system. The problem is often exacerbated by chemotherapy, which kills leucocytes (immune cells). Sometimes patients are unable to complete their chemotherapy treatment because their immune system has become dangerously weak, so it is very important to look for ways to overcome this problem.

In terms of Chinese medicine, the lungs are said to control immunity, the "defensive qi". However, the kidneys and digestion also play a role in supporting the immune system. When treating immune problems with acupuncture, it is essential to identify which organs need most support.

Researchers in Japan looked at concentrations of leucocytes (immune cells) before and after acupuncture. They found that, following acupuncture, there was a statistically significant increase in both the number of immune cells, and in certain key components of those cells. "These observations indicate that acupuncture may regulate the immune system and promote

---

29   Alimi D, *Journal of Clinical Oncology* 2003 Nov 15;21(22):4120–6.

the activities of humoral and cellular immunity as well as NK cell activity."[30] This is clear evidence that acupuncture can help maintain immunity.

One's state of mind has a profound impact on one's qi, and therefore by extension on one's immune system. This claim is supported by a study undertaken in America which explored whether acupuncture can help reverse reductions in immune cells caused by anxiety. Treatment was performed on 34 female patients, suffering from anxiety (as determined by the Beck Anxiety Inventory). Blood samples were taken before acupuncture, and 72 hours after it. A control group of 20 non anxious women was used. The researchers found that:

> Impaired immune functions in anxious women…were significantly improved by acupuncture and augmented immune parameters (superoxide anion levels and lymphoproliferation of the patient subgroup whose values had been too high) were significantly diminished. Acupuncture brought the above mentioned parameters to values closer to those of healthy controls, exerting a modulatory effect on the immune system.[31]

Several other studies have confirmed these findings,[32] suggesting that acupuncture has a significant role to play in supporting the immune system of cancer patients, particularly those undergoing chemotherapy.

---

30 Yamaguchi, N. *et al. Evidence Based Complementary and Alternative Medicine* 2007 Dec;4(4):447–53. The cells measured were CD2(+), CD4(+), CD8(+), CD11b(+), CD16(+), CD19(+), and CD56(+). The cellular components were IL-4, IL-1beta and IFN-gamma.

31 Arranz, L. *et al. American Journal of Chinese Medicine* 2007;35(1):35–51.

32 See for example the review of evidence conducted by Cohen *et al., Integrative Cancer Therapies* 4(2);2005.

Improved lung function

Breathlessness is a common problem in lung cancer, as well as in patients where the cancer has spread to the lymphatic system. Several studies have suggested that acupuncture may help to improve lung function.

A randomised control trial published in the *Lancet* looked at the effects of acupuncture in patients with chronic obstructive pulmonary disease. The researchers found that, after three weeks of treatment, "patients receiving traditional Chinese acupuncture reported significantly improved subjective breathlessness in addition to improved six minute walking distance."[33]

A team at the Royal Marsden Hospital in the UK looked at the effects of acupuncture on patients with breathlessness caused by cancer. It found improvements in respiratory rate, oxygen saturation and pulse rate. These were matched by the subjective improvements reported by the subjects, including a reduction in anxiety levels.[34] This study illustrates the effect acupuncture has on the whole person: not only did it help the symptoms being treated, it also helped the patients feel better in themselves.

One study suggested that the benefits of acupuncture in this area may be under-reported, because of the way literature searches are carried out: "Patients with severe chronic obstructive pulmonary disease may benefit from the use of acupuncture, acupressure, and muscle relaxation with breathing retraining to relieve dyspnea"...but "because of publication bias, trials on CAM modalities may not be found on routine literature searches."[35] Undoubtedly more high quality trials are needed, but we should also work harder to identify research which has already been done, and keep a more open mind about what kind

---

33   Jobst, K. *et al. Lancet* 1986;2:1416–19.

34   Filshie, J. *et al. Palliative Medicine* 1996;10:145–50.

35   Pax, C. *et al. Journal of Pain Symptom Management* 2000 Nov;20(5):374–87. CAM stands for Complementary and Alternative Medicine.

of research is valid. Because traditional acupuncture treatments are modified for each patient, based on traditional diagnosis including tongue and pulse, it is argued that one cannot aggregate the results of such treatments.

Western research methods also require that clinical trials are *replicable*. In other words, the trial must be conducted in such a way that other researchers are able to replicate the trial exactly. If the acupoints chosen vary according to the patient, this is obviously not possible in a strict sense. Exact replicability also deliberately excludes the role of the therapist, which Chinese medicine regards as part of the healing process. These kinds of research biases effectively invalidate most traditional acupuncture.

Moreover, in an attempt to comply with such research standards, there is the danger that a more standardised approach to treatment is adopted, which would mean that the benefits of treating the whole person are lost. There is also the danger that research trials are constructed which do not match what acupuncturists are actually doing in the community.

Treating xerostomia

Following the application of radiotherapy, the salivary glands may be damaged, resulting in a lack of salivation and a very dry mouth. Conventional medication, pilocarpine, is not always effective in treating this condition. The Radiation Oncology Service of the Naval Medical Center, San Diego, California, has been developing acupuncture techniques to treat this problem. They conducted a study of 50 patients suffering xerostomia following radiotherapy, using a set protocol of three needles in each ear, and one needle in each index finger. Salivation was measured using an XI (xerostomia inventory) index, which ranged from 0 to 25 points, 9 being classed as the normal median score. The study found that:

response (defined as improvement of 10% or better over base-line XI values) occurred in 35 patients (70%). Twenty-four patients (48%) have received benefit of 10 points or greater on the XI.[36]

The authors now recommend three to four weekly treatments followed by monthly sessions for most patients, although some patients achieve lasting response without further therapy. Several hospitals in the South West of England now use this protocol with cancer patients, obtaining similar results to the original study.[37]

The Department of Medicine in McMaster University, Canada, have developed a non-invasive method of stimulating the acupoints instead of using acupuncture needles, called Codetron. They used this technique to treat xerostomia in a study of 46 patients who had received radiotherapy to the head and neck area. They found that a statistically significant improvement occurred. This improvement was still in evidence six months after the treatment had been completed. A prospective randomised Phase III trial with appropriate controls is being planned. The study also noted that no complications occurred during the administration of the Codetron treatment, highlighting once again one of the benefits of acupuncture over drugs.[38]

Treating nausea and vomiting

Chemotherapy can induce this problem, which can be severely debilitating. Some patients stop chemotherapy because they are

---

36 Johnstone *et al. Cancer* 2002 Feb 15;94(4):1151–6. Copyright 2002 American Cancer Society.

37 Unpublished research obtained from visits to Derriford Hospital, Plymouth; Torbay Hospital; and Royal Devon and Exeter Foundation Trust.

38 Wong *et al. International Journal of Radiation Oncology, Biology, Physics* 2003 Oct 1;57(2):472–80.

unable to endure the nausea. Several patients have said to me that they would rather die than feel that ill. Conventional medicine is effective for some patients, but by no means all, so other forms of treatment are needed. The Cochrane Collaboration conducted a systematic review of the evidence for acupuncture's effectiveness in treating chemotherapy induced nausea and vomiting.[39] They looked at 11 trials, involving a range of acupuncture techniques (needles, electrical stimulation, magnets, and acupressure) and found that "acupuncture-point stimulation of all methods combined reduced the incidence of acute vomiting". Electro-acupuncture was most effective. The review also found that acupressure reduced acute nausea severity, and noted that "self-administered acupressure appears to have a protective effect for acute nausea and can readily be taught to patients". The main point used is Pericardium 6, discussed above. This point is located on the front of the forearm, near the wrist. It is between the two tendons (the tendons can be identified by clenching the hand into a fist). The patient finds the wrist crease, and then measures two thumb widths in the direction of the elbow.

Acupuncture can also treat postoperative nausea, which can cause problems after cancer surgery. One review found that "for postoperative nausea and vomiting, results from 26 trials showed acupuncture-point stimulation was effective for both nausea and vomiting". The author also looked at some of the possible mechanisms which could explain acupuncture's role in this area. He found that MRI scans showed that stimulation of Pericardium 6 induced "gastric myoelectrical activity, vagal modulation and cerebellar vestibular activities". In other words, the electrical activity of the stomach and the brain was stimulated by acupuncture.[40]

39   Ezzo, J. M. *et al. Cochrane Database Systematic Review* 2006 Apr 19;(2):CD002285.

40   Streitberger, K., *Autonomic neuroscience* 2006 Oct 30;129(1–2):107–17. Epub 2006 Sep.

Reducing hot flushes

Hot flushes can be a side effect of the drug Tamoxifen, which is used in women with breast cancer. Flushes are usually treated with HRT (hormone replacement therapy), but these drugs may increase the risk of certain cancers, and are therefore considered inappropriate for women with hormone sensitive carcinomas.

According to Chinese medicine, Tamoxifen tends to deplete the kidney yin (the cooling function). Acupuncture attempts to restore the yin, thereby controlling the hot flushes. HRT has a very cooling, dampening effect, which is why it can contribute to the development of certain cancers. The beauty of acupuncture is that it increases the yin, without causing cold or damp.

One study found acupuncture to be as effective at reducing hot flushes as estradol (the drug generally used). It was concluded that "acupuncture may be a safe alternative to those hormone replacement therapies with potentially adverse side effects".[41]

Two very recent studies by Beverly de Valois, at Thames Valley University, looked at the effectiveness of acupuncture for treating hot flushes caused by Tamoxifen and Arimidex. One study used a traditional approach, with treatments selected according to the individual presentation of the patient, and changing over time as appropriate. In this study, 48 women recorded an average reduction in hot flush frequency of 49.8 per cent over baseline. The women also showed improvements in other areas, such as mood, concentration, sexual behaviour, and sleep patterns.

The second study used a set protocol of ear acupuncture points (known as the "NADA Protocol"), and recorded an average reduction in hot flush frequency of 35.9 per cent. Improvements in other areas were also found in this study. One cannot draw

41   Wyon *et al. Climacteric* 2004;7:153–64.

very firm conclusions when comparing two groups of these sizes, but the studies suggest that the individualised treatments were more effective than the fixed protocol.[42]

Another study examined acupuncture in men who experienced hot flushes following castration for prostate cancer. It was found that 70 per cent of men reported fewer symptoms at 10 weeks, compared to baseline.[43]

These studies show that acupuncture may provide a good treatment option. However, the lack of control groups and small sample sizes point to the need for further large scale trials.

Surgery recovery

Surgery is often used with good effect to remove tumours. However, it often leaves patients feeling weak, and can also cause a range of other complications. Acupuncture can be used to prepare patients for surgery, and also to help them recover from it. Surgery often cuts the acupuncture meridians, which means that the flow of qi is impeded. Moreover, the qi flow is reduced in exactly those places where it needs to flow, to promote healing and minimise the risk of the cancer recurring. Acupuncture can help maintain the flow of qi following surgery.

In South Korea, medicinal plasters are commonly applied to acupoints for pain relief. The Department of Anesthesiology in Hanyang University Hospital, South Korea, undertook a study whereby a plaster soaked in capsicum was applied to the acupoint Stomach 36 (Zusanli in Chinese) following surgery for a hysterectomy. Ninety patients were assigned to one of three groups. The therapeutic group had the medicinal plaster applied

---

42 Beverley de Valois, unpublished PhD Thesis, Thames Valley University, research conducted at Lynda Jackson Macmillan Centre, Mount Vernon Cancer Centre, Northwood, Middlesex.

43 Hammar *et al. Journal of Urology* 1999;161:853–56.

to the correct acupoint. One control group had the *medicinal* plaster applied to a *non-acupoint*. The other control group had a *non-medicinal* plaster applied to the *acupoint*. None of the patients knew if they had the correct plaster, or if it was in the correct place.

The team found that those patients who had the medicinal plaster in the correct place needed significantly lower amounts of morphine than both control groups ($P < 0.01$). They concluded that "the incidence of postoperative side effects and the use of rescue anti-emetics [anti-nausea drugs] during the 72 hours after surgery were significantly reduced in group Zusanli compared with other groups".[44]

One acupuncture technique involves the insertion of tiny "interdermal needles", held in place by small plasters. A team from the Department of Anesthesiology, University of Hirosaki School of Medicine, Japan, investigated whether the use of these needles was helpful in reducing the complications of surgery. The results were published in the American Journal, *Anesthesiology*, in 2002. A total of 175 patients undergoing surgery were divided into two groups, one of which received the plasters, and a control group. The needles were inserted before surgery, and patients were asked to give scores on a variety of questions for four days after their operations. Those in the acupuncture group reported significantly lower pain, and "consumption of supplemental intravenous morphine was reduced 50 per cent, and the incidence of postoperative nausea was reduced 20–30 per cent in the acupuncture patients". The study also found that "plasma cortisol and epinephrine concentrations were reduced 30–50 per cent in the acupuncture group during recovery and on the first postoperative day". These chemicals are produced by the body in response to pain and stress, and can delay the healing

---

44   Kim, K. S. and Nam, Y. M., *Anesthesia and Analgesia* 2006 Sep;103(3):709–13.

process. Any technique which reduces their production will tend to speed recovery.[45]

Many patients find that their mobility is greatly restricted following surgery. Surgery is traumatic to the body, and often leaves areas of great tension and pain. This blocks the flow of qi, which is greatly needed for recovery, and also to help prevent recurrence of the cancer. One study applied acupuncture to 29 patients who had undergone surgery for breast cancer, and tested whether it helped their recovery. It was found that treatment improved the range of motion of the shoulder, as well as reducing tightness and heaviness in the arm, and reducing symptoms of lymph oedema.[46]

Acupuncture anaesthesia

One particularly exciting area for research is in the use of acupuncture as an alternative to general anaesthetic during surgery. When acupuncture is used in this way, postoperative recovery is usually quicker, and with fewer complications. Many western trained anaesthetists are exploring this method, and reporting their findings in the West. For example, a team from the Institute for Anaesthesiology, of the Dutch University of Nijmegen, went to China to observe the removal of thyroid adenomas (benign growths) from 20 patients using acupuncture anaesthesia. They reported that "postoperative recovery was rapid and complication free. Acupuncture anaesthesia did not provide complete analgesia, but was safe and preferable to general anaesthesia where there was a shortage of facilities".[47]

---

45   Kotani, N. *et al. Anesthesiology* 2001 Aug;95(2):349–56.
46   Alem *et al. Acupuncture in Medicine* 2008;26(2):86–93.
47   Kho, H. G. *et al. Anaesthesia* 1990 Jun;45(6):480–5.

Psychological and emotional support

We have seen already that acupuncture induces the production of opiates, which induce a state of relaxation and well-being. Such chemical changes help to deal with the range of emotions which inevitably accompany the diagnosis and treatment of cancer. Sometimes the emotion present may actually have contributed to the cancer, in which case it is especially important to treat it.

Pharmaceuticals tend to close down one's emotional life. Acupuncture, on the other hand, works to help people come to terms with their emotions, rather than just block them out. It can help people address negative emotional patterns which may have contributed to the development of the cancer. According to Chinese medicine, if negative emotions are not addressed, they will eventually cause physical problems. This is why drugs have side effects: one has merely pushed a mental imbalance into the physical level.

Thus, acupuncture helps stop negative *emotional* states causing problems in the *physical* organs. When one treats the emotion, one is also treating the organ associated with it. In Chinese medicine, emotions are normal, healthy aspects of human life. It is only when they become over-dominant that they become pathological, causing problems to the physical body.

In the chapter on cultivating the spirit, we saw that each negative emotion has an opposite, positive, state of mind. When this positive state is cultivated, alongside receiving acupuncture, powerful results can be achieved.

A cancer diagnosis can bring fear: fear for the future; fear of death; fear of what will happen to friends and family who rely on one. Fear is associated with the kidneys, and is treated by points on that meridian, such as Kidney 3. This point will also help to treat the shock of a cancer diagnosis.

Anger and frustration are associated with the liver, and cause the qi to stagnate. It is especially important to treat this, as we must keep the qi flowing in order to promote recovery. We can use Liver 3, "Great Rushing", to treat anger.

Hysteria, panic and anxiety are associated with the heart. These often occur following a cancer diagnosis, and may go on to cause insomnia, depression and other problems. We can use Heart 7, "Gate of the Spirit", to treat such problems.

Cancer can cause worry: about whether one will die, about how much one will suffer, about money, and about the people who may be left behind. It can cause the mind to go round in circles, in an unhelpful, obsessive way. This pattern is associated with the digestive system, and can cause problems with it, such as nausea, bloating and constipation. We can use a point such as Spleen 6 to treat this situation. This will treat both the emotional imbalance, as well as supporting digestive function.

Cancer can cause grief: one is facing the loss of loved ones, as well as the loss of one's own life. This emotion is associated with the lungs, and is treated by points such as Lung 9.

Of course, there are limits to what acupuncture can achieve with the emotions. As we have said, emotions are a normal and inevitable part of being human. However, we hope that, in combination with cultivating the spirit, we may be able to make them less overpowering, and help patients feel a fuller range of other emotions. Acupuncture patients will continue to feel grief, anxiety, anger and worry; but they may also be enabled to feel joy, peace and love.

Summary

We will conclude this section by quoting from a large study done on the benefits acupuncture offers to those with cancer:

Many individuals with cancer have turned to acupuncture because their symptoms persisted with conventional treatments, or as an alternative or complement to their ongoing treatments. Despite the immense popularity in the community, few large randomized trials have been conducted to determine the effects acupuncture has on cancer symptoms and side effects of treatments. A majority of the current studies have shown beneficial effects that warrant further investigation with large trial sizes.[48]

We should also note that this section has given but a sample of the kinds of conditions acupuncture can help with. Other problems commonly treated include fatigue, urinary and bowel dysfunction, radiation pneumonitis (lung damage), ulceration, menstrual disorders, and many others.

OTHER TECHNIQUES

Electro-acupuncture

This technique involves attaching electrodes to the head of the acupuncture needles, and passing a tiny electric current through them. It is widely used in China and the West by acupuncturists. We have mentioned a few studies already which looked at this technique, which can be stronger than conventional acupuncture for some conditions.

Traditional acupuncture causes the release of various opiate-like substances which help to control pain, but the use of electro-acupuncture (EA) can optimise this process. For example:

EA of 2 Hz accelerates the release of enkephalin, beta-endorphin and endomorphin, while that of 100 Hz selectively

---

48   Cohen *et al. Integrative Cancer Therapies* 2005;4(2):131–43.

increases the release of dynorphin. A combination of the two frequencies produces a simultaneous release of all four opioid peptides, resulting in a maximal therapeutic effect. This finding has been verified in clinical studies in patients with various kinds of chronic pain including low back pain and diabetic neuropathic pain.[49]

One study of three patients undertaken by doctors in the USA attempted to examine whether electro-acupuncture may enhance the effectiveness of chemotherapy. Meridians were identified which passed through the tumour, then needles were placed on the meridians, 1–2 cm proximal to the tumour. The positive electrodes were attached to these needles. Needles were also inserted on other points on the meridians, sited away from the tumour, on the arms or legs. The negative electrodes were attached to these needles. Electrical stimulation of 0.5–2 Hz was passed through the needles, for 25 minutes. The treatments were given 2–5 times per week, and patients continued to receive chemotherapy. The study found that the results were "significantly better than those that were expected", and that "acupuncture can be a useful modality to complement conventional cancer treatment and may potentiate the effects of chemotherapy". The authors plan to undertake another study with a larger sample of patients in a randomised controlled trial.[50] **NB: It must be stressed that this technique was performed under surgical conditions, and should not be attempted outside this context.**

In an even more radical approach, the Department of Thoracic Surgery, in the China–Japan Friendship Hospital, Beijing, have used electro-acupuncture directly to attack tumours in 320 patients, where the tumour was superficial enough

49   Han, J. S. *Neuroscience Letters* 2004 May 6;361(1–3):258–61.
50   Golianu, B. and Sebestyen, E. *Medical Acupuncture* 2004;17(1). Research undertaken 2002–2004.

to access. They inserted platinum electrodes directly into the tumour, and passed an electric current through them. They claim that in 123 cases complete remission was achieved, and in 129 cases partial remission was achieved.[51] While this research may not have been done according to western standards, it certainly seems to warrant further investigation. This technique may be used where a tumour is inoperable, or where the resources do not allow surgery as an option. **NB: It must be strongly emphasised that this is a surgical procedure, carried out in a hospital by very experienced doctors, and should in no way be attempted out of this context. To do so would be highly dangerous.**

Moxibustion

Moxibustion (moxa) is a technique that has been used for over 2000 years in China. It involves burning the herb Artemisia near acupoints. The chapter on herbal medicine explains that this herb has the properties of reducing blood stagnation, when taken internally. When burnt at acupoints it also has this effect, but can also be used to tonify the qi. Clinical experience has demonstrated that moxa can benefit the immune system, and several studies have supported this.

A comparative trial of 221 patients suffering from chemotherapy-induced leucopenia was undertaken in China, with patients being split into two groups. One group (113 patients) received moxa, and the other group (108 patients) received Chinese herbal medicine. In this trial, slices of ginger were placed over acupoints on the back, and the moxa placed on the slices and burnt (a common therapeutic method). After 10 days, those receiving "effective" treatment were 84.1 per cent in the moxa

---

51   Xin, Y. L. *et al. Zhongguo Zhong Xi Yi Jie He Za Zhi* 2001 Mar;21(3):174–6.

group, and 35.2 per cent in the herbal group. Fifteen days later, the therapeutic effects in the two groups were maintained.[52]

In a Japanese study, the proportions of different kinds of lymphocytes in the blood were found to have changed after the application of moxa, suggesting that moxa works by changing the kinds of immune cells produced.[53]

Another Japanese study showed that moxa also improved the function of platelets, thereby improving blood coagulation. The body's phagocytic function was also found to be enhanced.[54]

Several Japanese pharmacological studies have investigated the role of moxa in cancer management. One study found that the smoke has been found to induce DNA fragmentation of tumour cells; cause apoptosis of cancer cells ("cell suicide"); and scavenge free radicals. The authors of this study concluded that "these data demonstrate the antitumor potential of moxa smoke".[55] The anti-inflammatory effects of moxa were also noted.

Another study isolated key compounds of moxa, and demonstrated their anti-tumour activity against two kinds of oral carcinomas, one kind of salivary gland tumor, one kind of melanoma, and two kinds of leukaemia.[56]

SUMMARY

In this chapter we have shown that acupuncture has been used to treat all kinds of diseases in China for over 2000 years. Over

---

52 Zhao, X. X. *et al. Zhongguo Zhen Jiu* (Chinese journal, article in Chinese) 2007 Oct;27(10):715–20

53 Yamashita *et al. American Journal of Chinese Medicine* 2001;29(2):227–35.

54 Okazaki, M. *et al. American Journal of Chinese Medicine* 1990;18(1–2):77–85.

55 Sakagami, H. *In Vivo* 2005 Mar–Apr;19(2):391–7, and see 471–4.

56 Hatsukari, I. *et al. Anticancer Research* 2002 Sep–Oct;22(5):2777–82.

this time, huge expertise has been developed, both in diagnosis and treatment.

As well as treating the *symptoms* of cancer, and the *side effects* of conventional treatments, acupuncture aims to restore balance to the *whole person*. It makes a full diagnosis of the patterns involved, in order to restore the person to harmony of both body and mind.

Much of the research mentioned in this chapter clearly demonstrates the effectiveness of acupuncture in managing a range of problems associated with cancer. In addition, new forms of research are being developed which aim to capture the wider benefits acupuncture brings, in terms of treating the whole person. A research technique known as "whole systems research" (WSR) looks at the impact acupuncture has on the *whole system* of a person. WSR allows for flexibility in the acupuncture points selected, rather than prescribing set acupoints for each condition.

In addition, rather than trying to exclude the effect of the practitioner, WSR tries to incorporate it as a legitimate aspect of treatment. It recognises that the "bedside manner" of the therapist may influence the therapeutic outcome, and that it is better to allow for this, rather than trying to create an artificial situation where the practitioner is not allowed to speak to the patient.

Using this methodology, a study was constructed to analyse the effects of acupuncture on 45 patients receiving chemotherapy for breast cancer, over a 14-week period. A range of outcome measures were used (including a fatigue index, a quality of life index, and the Hospital Anxiety and Depression Scale) and measurements of medication were recorded. Semi-structured interviews were also used to gain further information. The study is ongoing, and offers great promise as a methodology which measures a complex intervention such as acupuncture.[57]

---

57   Price *et al. Integrative Cancer Therapies* 2006:5(4);308–14.

RESOURCES

If one is looking for a herbalist and an acupuncturist, it makes sense to see if one person can give both kinds of treatment. Most Chinese herbalists are also acupuncturists, but many acupuncturists are *not* Chinese herbalists. It therefore makes sense to look for a Chinese herbalist first, rather than an acupuncturist. However, in many areas in the West it is not possible to find a qualified Chinese herbalist, so we shall give details of acupuncture registers here. In any case, some patients may not be able or willing to take herbs.

United Kingdom

In the UK acupuncture is not regulated by law. However, it is strongly recommended that patients consult a member of the British Acupuncture Council, at www.acupuncture.org.uk. This website will allow you to find an acupuncturist in your area. Registered practitioners will have completed a first degree level training (although by no means an actual BA or BSc degree), and will be bound by a code of ethics.

United States

There is much variation between the different states: some require acupuncturists to belong to a register, while others do not. One needs to discover the position in one's own state.

There is also a national register of practitioners, the National Certification Commission for Acupuncture and Oriental Medicine (NCCAOM). This organisation has a website, which allows people to search for a registered practitioner in their area: www.nccaom.org. Some states require practitioners to be certified with this body.

Australia

There is a national register of acupuncturists: the Australian Acupuncture and Chinese Medicine Association (AACMA). This organisation has a website: www.acupuncture.org.au, which allows patients to find a practitioner in their area.

Acupuncturists in Victoria must be registered with the Chinese Medicine Registration Board of Victoria: www.cmrb.vic.gov.au. This website also has a practitioner search facility.

Canada

The position varies between provinces, with some regulating acupuncture, and others not doing so. The Chinese Medicine and Acupuncture Association of Canada has a website which allows one to find practitioners: www.cmaac.ca.

CHAPTER FOUR

Elixir of Life: Herbal Medicine in the Management of Cancer

CHAPTER CONTENTS

Introduction: an integrated approach • A brief history of Chinese herbal medicine and cancer • How a typical Chinese herbal formula for cancer is constructed • Herbs to treat the energetic pattern • Herbs to treat the side effects of chemotherapy, radiotherapy and surgery • Summary • Resources

INTRODUCTION: AN INTEGRATED APPROACH

The main thrust of the modern western approach to cancer involves using highly toxic chemicals to kill cancer cells, a treatment known as chemotherapy. Unfortunately chemotherapy is also very toxic to normal cells, and has serious side effects. Often, these side effects endanger the life of the patient, so the treatment has to be stopped.

Chemotherapy kills immune cells, so patients can die from infections that would not harm the average person. It poisons the liver, kidneys and heart. It kills the cells lining the digestive tract, preventing proper absorption of nutrients, making the patient very weak. In order to deal with these side effects, more chemicals are given, which in turn can have more side effects, requiring the use of yet more chemicals.

This is not to say that chemotherapy should never be used, but it is to say that a more balanced approach is needed. It is very interesting to visit a Chinese hospital, where cancer patients are given the option to receive herbal medicine to complement their chemotherapy, radiotherapy and surgery. The herbal doctors have access to the results of scans and blood tests, and are trained to take the results into account when prescribing herbs. Herbal formulae are constructed to nourish and support patients through their treatments; to minimise side effects; and to enhance the effectiveness of any drugs which are given. The Chinese take a very pragmatic approach to medicine: they use what works.

After several decades of clinical and pharmacological research, the Chinese have identified many herbs which are effective in treating the side effects of particular chemotherapy drugs. These herbs may be given alongside the drugs as a matter of course, in order to prevent side effects even occurring, rather than waiting for problems to manifest.

In addition, many herbs have been identified which help to kill cancer cells. One of the interesting results coming out of Chinese studies is that, unlike drugs, herbs are very selective in attacking cancer cells, and don't harm normal cells. Conversely, chemotherapy is highly toxic to normal cells as well as cancer cells. In fact, herbs usually have *positive* side effects, leaving patients feeling in better shape overall.

Several medical centres in the USA are now introducing a more integrated approach to cancer care, drawing on the Chinese model. Let us hope that this trend becomes more widespread.

We must state clearly that herbal medicine is a highly complex system, requiring many years to master. Incorrect use of herbs can make one's condition worse, and even be highly dangerous. Some people hold the mistaken view that because herbs are "natural" they are safe: the existence of many highly toxic plants should disabuse us of this notion. The purpose of this chapter is therefore definitely not to help patients self-medicate, rather, it is to help them understand in a general way how herbs are used; to explain how herbs can benefit those with cancer; and to help one find a good herbalist. It is also hoped that, through the presentation of evidence, the use of herbal medicine will become more widely accepted within mainstream healthcare settings.

A BRIEF HISTORY OF CHINESE HERBAL MEDICINE AND CANCER

History shows that herbs have long been considered to be in the front line of the fight against cancer in China. The earliest recorded book on Chinese medicine, the *Yellow Emperor's Internal Classic*, was written around 100 or 200 BC, and contains detailed descriptions of the following conditions:

- Dysphagia (ge zhong).

- Masses below the diaphragm cause by blood stasis (xia ge).

- Stone – like uterine masses (shi jia).

- Ovarian cysts/tumours (chang tan).

- Polyps (xi rou).

- Diaphragm obstructions (ge sai).

- Intestinal tumours (chang liu).

- Sinew tumours (jin liu).

We can see from this list how advanced Chinese physicians were in their knowledge of tumours. The book also discussed some of the causes of tumours, including qi stagnation, blood stagnation, excess cold or heat in the climate, and emotional factors. These factors allowed pathogens to accumulate, and tumours to develop. We looked at some of these patterns in the first chapter.

By the second century AD, cancer theory had made further advances. In the "Synopsis of the Golden Chamber" (c 150–219 AD) there are detailed descriptions of various cancers of the digestive system and of the uterus. A doctor called Hua Tuo (died 208 AD), who is known as the founder of surgery in China, wrote:

> When accumulations in the interior lead to illness and cannot be reached by needles or herbs, they must be cut out. First ask the patient to take Ma Fei San (Anaesthesia Boiling Powder). He will soon be intoxicated and lose consciousness. Then cut open the abdomen and dissect the intestines, wash with a herbal decoction, sew up the wound and cover with an anaesthetic paste. Four or five days later the pain will stop while the patient is still in a coma.[58]

The physician Li Gao (1180–1251) emphasised the importance of strengthening the *digestive qi* in the treatment of cancer, as well as attacking the tumour itself. We mentioned this principle in Chapter One, and shall see below that it is still closely followed in modern China. Li Gao's student Zhang Yuansu said that "a robust person will not suffer from accumulations, which is a condition affecting those who are deficient" (p.9). As we have seen, in terms of the Eight Principles, one must address the *deficiency*, as well as the *excess* part of the disease.

---

58   Li Peiwen (2003) *Management of Cance with Chinese Medicine.* St. Albans: Donica Publishing Ltd, p.3.

By the 14th century we have records of detailed herbal formulae being used.[59] Modern research has confirmed that many of the herbs in use then indeed have anti-cancer properties. Interestingly, doctors were well aware of the role of the emotions in the development of cancer:

When sorrow, anger and depression accumulate day and night, Digestive Qi[60] will be dispersed and dejected and Liver Qi forced into transverse counterflow. As a consequence, a concealed node will gradually form, as big as a counter in a game of go; the node will not be painful or itchy. Decades later, it will appear as a sunken sore known as ru yan (mammary rock).[61]

It was known that many tumours are caused by phlegm, and that phlegm in turn is caused by a weak digestive system. Great emphasis was therefore placed on the Digestive Qi. It was also known that liver qi stagnation was one of the main factors involved in the development of cancer.

---

59   The following formula was used by Dr Zhu Danxi:
        Da Huang (Radix et Rhizoma Rhei)
        Po Xiao (Mirabilitum Non-Purum)
        San Leng (Rhizoma Spargenii Stoloniferi)
        E Zhu (Rhizoma Curcumae)
        Shi Jian (Alkali Herbae)
        Tao Ren (Semen Persicae)
        Hong Hua (Flos Carthami Tintorii)
        Shui Zhi (Hirudo seu Whitmania)
        Nao Sha (Sal Ammoniacum)
        Bie Jia (Carapax Amydae Sinensis)
        Lai Fu Zi (Semen Raphani Sativi)
        Tian Nan Xing (Rhizoma Arisaematis)
        see Li Peiwen, p.9 (see Footnote 58).

60   Referred to in the text as "spleen qi", which we have noted is a poor translation of the original Chinese concept.

61   Dr Zhu Danxi, quoted in Li Peiwen, p.8 (see Footnote 58).

By the 17th century cancer theory had progressed much further still, and one sees many of the herbal formula being used which are still used today. There are many detailed descriptions of various kinds of cancer, such as that of Shen Douyan:

> At the initial stage, there is no sensation of cold, heat or pain; the affected area is purplish black in colour, but is not hard. Erosion occurs from the inside. The condition is caused by accumulation of Heat due to sexual intemperance after the age of 20 or Blood depletion and Qi Deficiency after the age of 40.[62]

"Sexual intemperance", in Chinese medicine, is said to deplete the kidney essence, and so weaken the body. Many physicians have emphasised the importance of strengthening the kidneys and the digestive system, a strategy known as "cultivating the root".

Since 1949, traditional methods have been complemented by modern pharmacological and clinical research. In China, doctors of herbal medicine specialise in certain areas, such as cancer, so there are many who have spent a lifetime working in this field. This gives them great depth of knowledge and experience. In Chinese hospitals, herbal medicine plays a key role in the integrated approach to cancer treatment.

We have selected only a few brief extracts from the extensive written records on the management of cancer with Chinese medicine. We can see from this material the gradual accumulation of a wealth of collective experience in China. Some in the West have criticised the "lack of evidence" for Chinese medicine: when analysing Chinese herbal treatments, one would do well to bear in mind the accumulated clinical experience of many centuries. By contrast, many pharmaceutical drugs have been tested for only a decade or two.

---

62   Li Peiwen, p.11 (see Footnote 58).

HOW A TYPICAL CHINESE HERBAL FORMULA FOR CANCER IS CONSTRUCTED

A formula will include different kinds of herbs, from the following categories:

Herbs to treat the energetic pattern

As we described in Chapter One, the first step is to make a diagnosis of the exact pattern involved. The Eight Principles are the cornerstone of such a diagnosis. Common patterns include:

- liver qi stagnation

- deficiency of digestive qi

- phlegm

- blood stagnation

- heat toxins

- deficiency of kidney yin, yang or essence.

Herbs will be selected to address each pattern.

Herbs selected according to modern pharmacological data

Much research has gone into placing solutions of herbs into cultures of cancer cells, to observe which are effective against different kinds of cancer. The next stage has been to isolate key active ingredients of herbs, in order to synthesise new drugs. Indeed, many drugs in common use today are already derived from plants. This approach has its merits, but also its limits. Herbs are complex chemical structures, which contain many compounds.

They have evolved over many millennia, in order to survive in often harsh conditions, and all the components of the plant are related to each other. The herb as a whole is therefore greater than the sum of its parts.

For example, within one herb, certain compounds neutralise the toxicity of other compounds. For this reason, using whole herbs is much less likely to cause side effects than using isolated compounds.

We know very little about many of the ingredients in most herbs, and we know even less about the synergistic actions of the various ingredients as they combine with each other. The synergy of the active compounds is further enhanced by the process of boiling the herb. When a herb is boiled, the ingredients combine together in complicated ways, which are hard to track even with modern research methods. To use any one compound in isolation may not capture the full potential of the herb.

The picture is further complicated when herbs are combined in formulae, because the various herbs in a formula work synergistically with each other. There is a huge amount of knowledge about how herbs can help each other work, or *potentiate* each other. When one multiplies the synergistic effects of a complex herbal formula, one begins to see how complex the chemical action of a herbal formula will be. Experienced practitioners will be aware of many synergistic actions of herb combinations, and know which herbs potentiate each other. Sometimes, certain herbs are also used to mitigate the side effects of other herbs, which may be toxic if used alone, but safe if prepared with certain other herbs.

We can begin to see how modern research protocols can not measure the full effects of traditional Chinese herbal medicine. Modern protocols call for a clearly identified, standardised substance to be administered to a large number of people. They also require a "control group" who do not receive the set substance. However, traditional Chinese herbal medicine does not work in this way: because herbs are selected according to the energetic pattern of the patient, the formula will vary according to the patient. Herbal formulae cannot therefore be standardised across large groups. Indeed, the same formula is never given even to two people. Nevertheless, pharmacological data do have their place, if used in the wider context of traditional Chinese herbal medicine.

Herbs selected to treat the side effects of surgery, chemo- or radiotherapy

We will look at some approaches in this key area in more detail below. Orthodox medicine tends to focus on the removal of the tumour itself, rather than on helping the patient return to balance. There is certainly a place for this aspect, and the Chinese have a saying that "one needs to use a toxin to treat a toxin". We have also seen that they have practiced surgery to remove tumours since at least the second century. In terms of the Eight Principles, conventional medicine is removing the *excess*, but it is not addressing the *deficiency* of the patient. In the process of attacking the tumour, therefore, western medicine may actually worsen any energetic imbalance the patent has. This may manifest as side effects, such as nausea, insomnia, fatigue, lowered immunity, emotional problems, and organ damage. By addressing the deficiency aspect of the patient, herbal medicine can help people through the difficult orthodox treatment.

Herbs selected for the mental–emotional aspects

In Chinese medicine, each organ is associated with a specific mental–emotional state, and these states often contribute to the development of cancer. Being given a cancer diagnosis often makes the situation worse. Conventional treatments may also further exacerbate any problems, by weakening the body's qi, and having a negative impact on the mind. So, it is very important to address such issues, and we shall mention a few examples of herbs used in this way.

Grief affects the lungs, and we treat this using a certain kind of lily bulb (Lilium brownii, bai he). Irritability and over-excitement affect the heart, and are often treated with wild date seed (Ziziphus jujube/spinoza, suan zao ren). This herb also promotes restful sleep. It contains a compound called jujuboside, which has a sedative effect. Caution should be used with this herb when taken alongside barbiturates, as it potentiates their effect (that is, it makes them work more strongly).[63]

Anger affects the liver, and in this case we can use a herb such as Szechuan lovage (Ligusticum, chuan xiong). Chemically speaking, the herb is also a sedative, and in Chinese medicine is said to soothe the liver. This herb is often used with cancer, as it promotes qi and blood circulation (it is an anti-coagulant, and is used to treat thrombosis[64]).

Worry affects the digestion, and for this we can use longan berries (Euphoria longan, long yan rou). This herb has a very calming affect, and helps with the worry that inevitably accompanies cancer.

So, a variety of herbs will be selected, according to the presenting pattern of the patient. In China a typical cancer formula may consist of 15 to 20 herbs. The daily dose may be around 200 grammes (about eight ounces), which is very high by western

---

63   Chen, J. and Chen, T. (2000) *Chinese Medicine Herbology and Pharmacology.* City of Industry, CA: Art of Medicine Press, p.764.

64   Chen, J. and Chen, T. (2000) *Chinese Medicine Herbology and Pharmacology.* City of Industry, CA: Art of Medicine Press, p.616.

standards. Usually western people are unable to take such large formulae, and the dose here may be half or less of the Chinese one.

The traditional Chinese method of taking herbs is to boil them up every day in a pan (it is possible to take herbs in other ways, see below in "what kind of herbs take").

Patients may take herbs for many months, or even years, until they have returned to full health. If patients are taking herbs for long periods, they may be switched to capsules or tablets.

Now that we have looked at some of the general principles of constructing Chinese herbal formulae for cancer, let us look in more detail at some of the key herbs used.

HERBS TO TREAT THE ENERGETIC PATTERN

As we have mentioned above, a diagnosis must first be made. Once this is done, appropriate herbs can be selected from each category. In Chinese herbal medicine, herbs are organised according to energetic categories. Some of the most common categories that are used with cancer are as follows:

- Herbs to nourish the digestive qi.

- Herbs to break up phlegm.

- Herbs to move liver qi stagnation.

- Herbs to break up blood stagnation.

- Herbs to clear heat toxins.

- Herbs to nourish the kidneys.

In this section we shall look at some of the key herbs in each of these categories, and how they are used in the management of cancer. Within each category, certain herbs have been identified which are particularly useful in working with cancer.

There is a great amount of knowledge about the energetic properties of herbs, which has been synthesised over many centuries. Herbs are classified according to their thermal nature, into hot, warm, neutral, cool and cold. In western terms, a "hot" herb will have a stimulating effect on the metabolism, whereas a "cold" herb will tend to slow the metabolism down, and have more of a sedating effect. When working with cancer one tends to use herbs which are neutral or warm, as these are more suited to the nature of the human person: we are seen as slightly warm.

Herbs are also classified according to which organ they "enter". As with any substance ingested, herbs tend to have effects on particular parts of the body. Certain herbs are sometimes used as "messenger herbs", because they take the other herbs to a certain part of the body. For example, the herb jie geng is said to go to the throat, so if one wants to focus on the throat, one adds this herb to the formula. Herbs may enter more than one organ: liquorice for example enters all 12 main organs. This is why this herb is used so frequently in Chinese herbal medicine, because it has a general harmonising effect. It is known to mitigate the harsh properties of many herbs, and modern research has shown that it neutralises many toxins.

Herbs are classified according to whether they are tonifying or clearing. In western terms, "tonifying" herbs tend to contain high levels of nutrients, while "clearing" herbs tend to contain chemicals which fight micro-organisms, or which help break down toxins, such as cholesterol for example.

The emphasis is placed on tonifying, rather than on clearing, in patients with cancer. Herbs are therefore selected which have a gentle nature. One tends to avoid herbs which are too cold in nature, as they weaken the digestive qi and the kidneys.

One also avoids using too many herbs which are very moving or dispersing in nature, because they can disturb the normal flow of qi and blood. This focus is especially necessary in modern cancer care, as conventional treatments are quite clearing and harsh in nature.

We must strongly emphasise that the herbs we are about to discuss must not be selected by those who are not experienced practitioners of Chinese herbal medicine. We are discussing these herbs as examples only. As we have said, herbs must be selected following a detailed diagnosis, and a formula created which meets the exact energetic pattern of the patient. If the wrong herbs are selected, they may well make the situation worse. Herbs are powerful substances, which can cause great harm if used improperly.

Herbs to nourish the digestive qi

We have seen how important it is to strengthen the digestive system. The digestive system produces qi and blood, but when it is weak food turns into phlegm. Weakness of the digestive qi is often one of the main underlying patterns leading to the development of cancer. This weakness may be further exacerbated by the worry of receiving a cancer diagnosis. In addition, chemotherapy can weaken the digestive system still further. Those receiving chemotherapy are very often nauseous, which is a sign that the digestive qi has been weakened. Herbs from this category usually play a prominent role in cancer formulae.

One of the most important herbs in this category is Astragalus (huang qi). This herb strengthens the qi of the digestive system and the lungs. According to traditional Chinese medicine, Astragalus strengthens the defensive qi of the body, and modern research confirms that the herb indeed boosts the immune system. A group of research institutions looked at the effects of using Astragalus to support platinum based chemotherapy, and made a meta analysis of 34 randomised trials, covering a total of 2815 patients. They found that Astragalus increased the effectiveness of the treatment, and helped patients to live longer, concluding that "Astragalus-based Chinese herbal medicine may increase effectiveness of platinum-based chemotherapy".[65] The study concluded that "Astragalus has been shown to have immunologic benefits by stimulating macrophage and natural killer cell activity and inhibiting T-helper cell type 2 cytokines". In other words, the herb encourages the body to produce cells which fight the cancer cells.

Another herb which is used to strengthen the digestion is a fungus known as Poria (fu ling). By strengthening the digestion, this herb also helps to remove phlegm from the body (remember that in Chinese medicine phlegm is produced when the digestive qi fails to break food down properly). This herb has long been used to treat phlegm based cancers in Chinese medicine. The Chinese University of Hong Kong undertook to investigate the action of Poria, and placed a substance derived from the herb in test tubes with breast cancer cells.[66] They found that "cancer-cell growth was decreased by 50 per cent of the control level". The study found that the substance induced apoptosis (cell death)[67] in the cancer cells.[68] We should note that the substance concerned is water soluble, that is, it is extracted into water. We will discuss below the issue of using herbal tinctures (herbs which are extracted into alcohol), suffice to note for now that the active ingredient may not be extracted in the same way into alcohol, so

---

65   *Journal of Clinical Oncology* 2006;24(3):419–30.

66   The substance was the polysaccharide beta-glucan PCM3–II.

67   Apoptosis is the process whereby cells kill themselves. Cells are programmed to do this, and cancers often form when this fails to occur.

68   *Oncology Reports* 2006 Mar;15(3):637–43.

one cannot assume that a tincture of the herb has the same effect as a decoction (boiling the herb in water).

Another herb which is used to support the digestive system and clear phlegm is "Job's tears" (Coix lacryma-jobi, in Chinese yi yi ren). There are written records of this herb being used in the second century.[69] The plant is a relative of maize, and a staple part of the diet in South East China. It had long been observed that those living in the area had low rates of cancers, and a pharmacologist Li Dapeng believed that this was due to the consumption of Jobs tears. In 1975 he started work to try and identify which part of the plant had anti-tumour properties, and 20 years later he had produced a drug called Kanglaite based on a key compound contained in the herb. The drug has been administered to several hundred thousand people in China, and in 2003 was given Stage Two approval by the Food and Drug Administration (FDA) in the United States for clinical trails with patients with non-small cell lung cancer.[70]

Herbs to break up phlegm

We have noted that herbs which strengthen the digestive qi also play a role in helping to reduce and prevent the formation of phlegm. However, there are herbs which have a much stronger effect in directly clearing phlegm. These herbs will often cause people to expectorate a lot of phlegm during their treatment. These herbs are particularly appropriate in those kinds of cancers which are caused by phlegm.

The loquat leaf (pi pa ye; Eriobotrya japonica) is a herb which is said to break up phlegm in the lung and stomach, and is therefore indicated in the management of phlegm based cancers

---

69 In the Divine Husbandman's Classic of the Materia Medica, Shen Nong Ben Cao Jing, cited in Chen and Chen (2004) p.390 (see Footnote 63).

70 *Science* 10 January 2003;299.

in those organs. A study by Okayama University in Japan, published in the United States, discovered that certain compounds in the herb had significant anti-tumour activity.[71]

Herbs to move liver qi stagnation

This pathology can cause the accumulation of toxins, and also blood stagnation. Inevitably cancer will involve some degree of stagnation, and it is important to address this factor. The liver channel goes through the breast, and is often indicated in breast cancer. We mentioned above the herb Szechuan lovage which can be used to treat this imbalance.

Herbs to break up blood stagnation

Many kinds of tumours are caused by blood stagnation. However, one does not generally use too many of these herbs over an extended period, as they can disrupt the normal flow of qi and weaken the patient. In any case, by attacking the tumour conventional treatments treat the blood stagnation itself, so the herbal formula can focus more on the underlying weaknesses. In other words, the orthodox treatment focuses on the *excess* (the tumour), while the herbal treatment focuses on the *deficiency*.

With cancer, one often uses herbs which have a gentle effect in moving the blood, rather than herbs which have a forcible effect of breaking up blood stagnation. This strategy helps to prevent the blood becoming stagnant again, after a tumour has been removed. One herb used in this way is Angelica sinensis (dang gui), which gently moves the blood, and also nourishes the blood, making it a gentle herb suitable for cancer formulae. One study undertaken in the University of Minnesota has

---

71   *Journal of Agricultural and Food Chemistry* 2002 Apr 10;50(8):2400–3.

shown that Angelica may be helpful with prostate cancer. A compound isolated from the herb called "decursin" interferes with the androgen signalling pathways which are crucial for the development of some prostate cancers. Decursin also induces apoptosis in prostate cancer cells. Decursin was found to be "more potent than bicalutamide for suppressing androgen-stimulated cell growth".[72] (Bicalutamide, brand name Casodex, is the drug which is currently used for this purpose.) It is important to note that it is an *isolated compound* which is effective, and one can not assume that the raw herb itself will have the same effects as the compound. Nevertheless, this study helps to justify the historical use of Angelica in the treatment of prostate cancer.

The Chinese herb tao ren (Prunus persica, or common peach seed) has been used since the fourteenth century for certain kinds of tumours. This herb is known to act strongly to break up blood stagnation, and is much stronger than a herb such as Angelica. Indeed it has long been known to be toxic if taken in too high a dose, which is confirmed by modern pharmacological research, as well as by known cases of overdose. Peach seeds contain several compounds which seem to have an anti-tumour activity, among which are amygdalin and prunasin. A study by Okayama University in Japan, which tested the herb both in vitro (in test tubes) and in vivo (in live animals) found that amygdalin and prunasin had significant anti-tumour activity.[73] The compounds were also found to be effective against the activity of the Epstein–Barr virus.

There are several Chinese herbs which contain the compound curcumin, and "pharmacological studies have demonstrated that curcumin from Curcuma longa is an antimutagen as well as an antipromotor for cancer".[74] Curcuma longa (jiang

72   *Molecular Cancer Therapy* 2007 Mar;6(3):907–17.

73   *Biological and Pharmaceutical Bulletin* 2003 Feb;26(2):271–3.

74   Han, R. *Stem Cells* 1994 Jan;12(1):53–63.

huang) is turmeric, and has long been used to break up tumours caused by blood stagnation, especially in the digestive organs and the liver. Curcumin is also found in the herb yu jin (Radix curcuma), which has a similar function of breaking blood stagnation, but is said to work on the heart, liver and gall bladder. Curcumin is also found in the herb e zhu (Rhizome curcuma), which is said to treat the digestion and liver organs. This herb is commonly given intravenously in China to cancer patients, and is particularly indicated for cervical carcinoma.[75] This supports the traditional understanding that the herb clears stagnation from the liver channel, as the liver channel runs through the cervix.

Herbs to clear heat toxins

Heat toxins can be a major contributory factor in the development of cancer. Many herbs have traditionally been used to treat this imbalance, and modern pharmacological research is confirming that certain compounds in these herbs indeed have anti-tumour actions. One such herb is the leaves from isatis/indigo woad (Da Qing Ye). This herb is used to clear heat toxins from the heart, stomach and lung, and is used to treat febrile disorders such as measles, meningitis, encephalitis, mumps and scarlet fever, as well as jaundice. The compound Indirubin, contained in the herbs, "is useful for the treatment of chronic myelocytic leukaemia".[76]

Herbs to nourish the yin

The yin is the cooling, calming, nourishing energy in the body. A deficiency of the yin can lead to overheating, and a lack of

---

75   The herb has shown promising results against cervical tumours in mice, see Chen and Chen, p.667 (see Footnote 63).

76   Han, R. *Stem Cells* 1994 Jan;12(1):53–63.

moisture and nourishment in the body. This can be a contributory factor in certain kinds of cancer. One herb which as traditionally been used to nourish the yin, especially the yin of the liver, is Artemesia annua (Qing Hao, sweet wormwood). This herb is particularly effective when the patient has a deficiency of yin, and also has heat toxins. It is used to treat jaundice, febrile disorders, and certain menopausal symptoms. One particularly important use of the herb is to fight malaria. Pharmacological research has shown that the compound Artesunate, synthesised from the herb, contains compounds which "target several proteins in Plasmodia, which is thought to result in killing of the micro-organism" (Plasmodia are the micro-organisms which transmit malaria). Artesunate also causes apoptosis and necrosis in cancer cells.[77]

Focus on some common cancers

PROSTATE CANCER

In Chinese medicine there are a number of factors which may be involved in the development of this cancer. The digestive qi is often weak, leading to the build up of phlegm. This situation maybe exacerbated by the consumption of too much greasy food, which cannot be digested properly. The kidney yang may be weak, and in Chinese medicine the kidney yang is responsible for clearing phlegm and heat toxins from the lower abdomen. Stagnation of liver qi may also be present, which can be caused by emotional problems or stress. This can then lead to blood stagnation. Eventually, the above factors lead to the accumulation of heat toxins, phlegm, and blood stagnation around the prostate, which contributes to cancer there. As with all cancers, it is important to identify the proportions in which each

---

77   Li, P. C. *et al. Cancer Research* 2008 Jun 1;68(11):4347–51.

of the pathogens is present. In some patients, one will need to focus more on clearing phlegm, while in others one will need to focus more on clearing blood stagnation, for example. There are recognised herbal base formulae for each of the main patterns mentioned, but these must be carefully modified for each patient.[78]

In 1996 a product called PC SPES was developed and marketed for the treatment of prostate cancer. It contained a mixture of eight herbs (discussed below) in capsules, each of which seems to have some anti-tumour effect. This product moved away from the traditional method of designing a formula for each patient, in an attempt to come up with a standard formula which could be used for all cases of prostate cancer. One advantage of this approach is that a diagnosis does not need to be made, thus saving resources. Another advantage is that research trials of a fixed substance can be undertaken, and the results aggregated.

One such trial showed that all 33 participants who had androgen *dependent* prostate cancer experienced a fall in their PSA level of over 80 per cent (PSA is a measure of the activity of the cancer), and 19 out of the 37 with androgen *independent* prostate cancer had a fall of over 50 per cent in their PSA.[79] In 2002 PC SPES was withdrawn due to concerns over contaminants, but PC SPES2 was developed by Active Botanicals (UK Ltd), and rigorously tested to exclude contaminants before being launched. One month into treatment, seven out of ten patients had a fall in their PSA doubling time.[80] The authors concluded that "PC-SPES2 offers renewed hope and a safe alternative treatment option for patients with ad-

---

78   Li Peiwen, pp.540–3 (see Footnote 58).

79   *Journal of Clinical Oncology* 2000 Nov 1;18(21):3595–603.

80   *Oncology Reports* 2008 Mar;19(3):831–5.

vanced HRPC.[81] Further investigation with phase II trials is warranted".

Both of the PC SPES trials observed that a significant number of patients withdrew from the study because of severe diarrhoea. This is exactly what a practitioner of Chinese medicine would expect with such a formula. The herbs in PC SPES are ones which clear heat toxins, and are therefore very "cold" in nature. Very cold herbs tend to weaken the digestion. Patients with cancer often have weak digestive systems anyway, so such a formula could weaken them still further. We have seen that herbal formulae for cancer emphasise *strengthening* the system, not just clearing toxins. If a patient had a weak digestive system, a Chinese herbalist would add herbs to strengthen the digestive system and prevent diarrhoea. If this is not done, the formula may help to clear the cancer in the short term, but by weakening the system could cause problems in the long term. Thus we can see the limitations of the approach of using a fixed formula to treat all patients. With properly individualised formulae, one would hope to avoid the side effects seen with PC SPES.

Let us take a look at the herbs in PC SPES:

- Chrysanthemum morifolium (ju hua): clears heat toxins, especially from the liver.

- Isatis indigota (da qing ye): we mentioned this herb above, which clears heat toxins, and has anti-tumour actions.[82]

- Panax pseudoginseng (San qi): disperses blood stagnation, which is a major contributory factor in many cancers.

---

81   HRPC is Hormone Refactory Prostate Cancer. This is prostate cancer which does not respond to conventional hormonal treatment, and is therefore very hard to treat.

82   This herb contains indirubin which has been shown to have an inhibiting effect on leukaemia, sarcoma and lung cancer in mice.

- Rabdosia rubescens (dong ling cao): clears heat toxins, and has anti-tumour activity.[83]

- Scutellaria baicalensis (huang qin): clears heat toxins.

- Ganoderma lucidum (ling zhi): this is a fungus which supports the qi. It herb has been shown to have anti-tumour activity, by causing an increase of various immune cells.[84]

- Glycyrrhiza glabra (gan cao, liquorice): supports the qi, especially of the digestive system, and has a gentle, moderating effect. It is often used to moderate the harsh actions of toxin-clearing herbs.

- Serenoa repends (Saw Palmeto): this is a western herb used for prostate problems. Its use here is a good example of combining Chinese and western herbs.

As we noted above, this formula contains mostly herbs which clear heat toxins. These are herbs which directly attack the cancer itself, rather than supporting the qi of the person. If a patient with weak qi was to take PC SPES, one would prescribe herbs to strengthen the qi alongside it.

LUNG CANCER

In Chinese medicine it has long been recognised that one of the most important factors in lung cancer is "invasion of heat toxins". This includes environmental pollution and, in modern society, cigarette smoke. The heat toxins dry out the lung yin, so the tissues are not nourished properly. The heat toxins

---

83   The injection of the compound rubescensine A, isolated from the herb, has been shown to inhibit esophageal and liver cancer in mice and rats. *Chinese Herbal Pharmacology Journal* 1986;(4):361.

84   *International Journal of Cancer* 1997 Mar 17;70(6):699–705.

also weaken the qi of the lungs, which leads to the accumulation of phlegm. The weak lung qi also causes the qi to stagnate, which in turn causes blood stagnation. Emotional factors are often involved, and in Chinese medicine we say that grief injures the lungs. Lung cancer often develops after the loss of a loved one.

Around 80 per cent of lung cancers are "non-small cell lung carcinomas" (NSCLC), which do not respond well to chemotherapy. With advanced NSCLC, the prognosis is very poor. In 1991, Beijing Hospital of Traditional Chinese Medicine decided to construct a trial to see whether Chinese herbs could help in the fight against this disease.[85] They divided a group of 136 patients with advanced NSCLC into three groups. One group was given chemotherapy alone, one group was given Chinese herbs alone, and one group was given Chinese herbs plus chemotherapy. It was found that the administration of the herbs increased the responsiveness of patients to the chemotherapy: those who received chemotherapy alone had a 27.2 per cent response rate, while those who received chemotherapy plus herbs had a response rate of 44.4 per cent.

It was also found that those receiving herbs had a lower rate of side effects, such as coughing, sputum, fatigue, and breathlessness. They also reported a better quality of life.

Perhaps most interestingly, it was found that life expectancy was highest in the group which received herbs plus chemotherapy (see table, p.158).

---

85 Yang Guo-wang, Wang Xiao-min, Han Dong *et al.* Beijing Hospital of Traditional Chinese Medicine, Beijing 100010, "Study on TCM comprehensive therapy in the treatment of advanced non-small cell lung cancer"; first published in *China TCM Information Journal* 2005;(12):11, translated into English by Zhong Zhi Chen, Beijing Univeristy of Traditional Chinese Medicine.

Survival rates after chemotherapy and herbal treatment

	One-year survival rates	Average survival time
Chemotherapy alone	27.3%	9.2 months
Herbs alone	36.1%	11.5 months
Chemotherapy plus herbs	48.9%	12.3 months

Comparable patients who received no treatment would have been expected to survive around four to six months.

This kind of cancer is very hard to treat with conventional methods, and with such cancers there seems to be an especially important role for Chinese herbal medicine.

In order to match western research methods, in many clinical trials patients are given *set* formulae, rather than allowing the practitioner to design a formula for each patient, in the traditional Chinese way. Conversely, one of the positive aspects of this trial on lung cancer, from a Chinese perspective, was that the formulae were modified according to the presenting Chinese medicine diagnosis.[86]

---

86   A methodology was developed as a compromise between having a fixed formula, and allowing physicians to select herbs completely at random. Set herbs (three or four for each category) were added when the following patterns were present in the patient:
   • Yin deficiency.
   • Qi deficiency.
   • Phlegm.
   • Blood stagnation.
   • Toxic heat.
   • Yang deficiency.
   • Blood deficiency.

BREAST CANCER

This is the most common form of cancer in western non-smoking women. It appears to be much more prevalent in the West: in the United Kingdom, around 75 women per 100,000 develop breast cancer; in China the figure is only about 16. The higher figure in the UK may partly be explained by better detection rates, and because the population lives longer on average (older people are more likely to get cancer). However, from the perspective of Chinese medicine, it seems likely that a western diet, high in fats and sugar, would also be a contributory factor. The high levels of stress may also play a part, and this may be exacerbated by the lack of support in many people's lives in the West. One thing that I noticed in Chinese oncology units was the amount of family members that accompanied relatives with cancer to hospital. In the inpatients department, there would often be several relatives sitting with the patient for many hours, often having brought them food. This stands in marked contrast to the situation in the West.

In Chinese medicine, high stress levels affect the liver, and one of the main contributory factors to breast cancer is liver qi stagnation. The liver channel runs through the breast, and so stagnation in the liver can cause a build up of phlegm, heat toxins and blood stagnation there.

Liver qi stagnation is also caused by anger and frustration, so these may also play a role in the development of breast cancer. This was discussed in the chapter on cultivating the spirit.

When liver qi stagnation is a factor in her breast cancer, the patient will often feel a sense of oppression, pressure or tightness in the chest. She may suffer from depression, anger, irritability, headaches, or breast distension. Often, these problems are worse just before menstruation.

Another factor which often contributes to breast cancer is weakness in the digestive system, causing a build up of phlegm.

Digestive deficiency may also cause tiredness and a general lack of qi, exacerbating the problem. The stomach meridian runs through the breast, so problems in that organ may cause stagnation in the breast area, particularly a build up of phlegm there. One of the most common base formulae for breast cancer is called "Free and Easy Wanderer" (xiao yao san). This formula is named after the Taoist sage, Chuang Tsu, who we discussed in the chapter on cultivating the spirit. He lived a carefree existence, wandering around China meeting weird and wonderful people. He cultivated an attitude of detachment to the problems of the world, mixed with a fine sense of humour.

Herbs often help people on a mental level, as well as on a physical one: this formula can help people to feel more relaxed and less tense. However, one must also work to cultivate this state of mind in order to bring about deep and steady changes to one's mental outlook. Herbs can be like teachers, showing us new ways of being, but it is up to us to integrate their lessons into our daily lives.

Many women who have had breast cancer will be put on drugs to block oestrogen, such as Tamoxifen. Oestrogen is considered to be a yin hormone, as it is cold and damp in nature. Too much oestrogen can therefore contribute to the formation of damp and phlegm, and lead to breast tumours. By blocking the oestrogen, Tamoxifen reduces the amount of phlegm in the breast, and so makes tumours less likely. However, by blocking the yin, it is likely that the patient may become yin deficient. This can lead to too much heat, and symptoms such as hot sweats, which are indeed a common side effect of Tamoxifen. Chinese herbs can therefore be used to nourish the yin, and counter the side effects of Tamoxifen.

We must emphasis again that it is important to use herbs according to a precise energetic diagnosis. A skilled practitioner needs to judge the correct amount of yin tonics needed in any given case: too many may lead to an increase of phlegm, and is therefore contra-indicated, because it was phlegm which contributed to the original cancer. The practitioner will need to monitor the patient carefully, to ensure that signs of phlegm do not start showing. One of the skills of the herbalist is to know just when to stop administering each herb.

LIVER CANCER

Many cancers of the liver arise in patients with liver cirrhosis, in whom their incidence is high. In Chinese medicine we say that these people have heat toxins in the liver. A traditional formula which helps this pattern is known as "Minor Bupleurum Decoction" (Xiao Chai Hu Tang in Chinese, Sho-saiko-to in Japanese). Researchers in the Osaka City University Medical School, Japan, conducted a randomised trial on 260 patients with cirrhosis. Half of the patients were given the formula, and half were not. After five years, the incidence of liver cancer was statistically less in the group taking the herbs, which also had higher survival rates.[87]

The formula contains seven herbs. It has herbs to clear liver heat toxins (bupleurum and scutellaria), and herbs to clear phlegm (pinellia and ginger). As well as these *clearing* herbs, the formula also contains herbs to *tonify* the qi and blood (ginseng, black dates and liquorice), which is vital in cancer formulae. The formula is therefore very balanced, clearing toxins and phlegm, but also nourishing the qi and blood.

It is interesting to note that the dose is very low by modern Chinese standards. Japanese herbal medicine, called Kampo, tends to use much lower doses than modern Chinese herbal medicine. Kampo also tends to stick more closely to classical formulae, such as this one, mentioned in the *Shan Han Lun* (written

---

87   Oka, H. *et al. Cancer* 1995 Sep 1;76(5):743–9.

around 220 AD). In modern China, most doctors tend to design their own formulae, which are often 200 grammes per day. In this trial the dose was only 7.5 grammes per day.

HERBS TO TREAT THE SIDE EFFECTS OF CHEMOTHERAPY, RADIOTHERAPY AND SURGERY

Herbal medicine has been used for many decades in Chinese hospitals to treat the side effects of western cancer treatments. It has been estimated that up to 60 per cent of patients undergoing these therapies suffer some kind of side effects.[88] Orthodox treatments can reduce immunity, induce severe nausea and fatigue, and induce a general feeling of low mood and malaise. Chinese herbs can be very effective in dealing with such side effects, and in helping patients to complete their conventional treatments.

Strengthening immunity

Chemotherapy can drastically impair the immune system, by causing a reduction in the production of lymphocytes (immune system cells). Sometimes this reduction becomes so dangerous that the treatment cannot be completed. In such cases, the administration of herbs can allow patients to complete a treatment, which they may otherwise have been unable to do.

---

88   Zhang, M., Liu, X., Li, J., He, L. and Tripathy D. "Chinese medicinal herbs to treat the side-effects of chemotherapy in breast cancer patients". *Cochrane Database of Systematic Reviews* 2007, Issue 2. Art. No.: CD004921. DOI: 10.1002/14651858.CD004921.pub2.

The Cochrane Collaboration[89] has investigated the use of Chinese herbs to counter the side effects of chemotherapy in patients with breast cancer. They identified seven randomised controlled trials, involving 542 breast cancer patients, and concluded that:

> using Chinese herbs in conjunction with chemotherapy or CHM [Chinese Herbal Medicine] alone may be beneficial in terms of improvement in marrow suppression and immune system, and may improve overall state of quality of life.[90]

The Cochrane Collaboration has also investigated the use of Huang Qi (Astagalus, mentioned above) in patients undergoing chemotherapy for colorectal cancer. It found that:

> Compared with patients treated by chemotherapy alone, patients treated with chemotherapy and Huangqi decoctions were less likely to experience nausea and vomiting or low white cell counts. There was some evidence to suggest that the decoctions also stimulated cells of the immune system, but did not affect the levels of antibodies in the blood. We could find no evidence of harm arising from the use of Huangqi decoctions. Our results suggest that further, larger-scale, trials of the use of Huangqi decoctions in the prevention of chemotherapy-related side-effects are needed.[91]

Scientists at the University of California have synthesised a drug from huang qi, called TAT2, which enhances the activity

---

89   The Cochrane Collaboration is an independent organisation which examines evidence for various medical treatments. It is recognised to be impartial and of the very highest standard.

90   Cited above, Zhang *et al.* (see Footnote 88).

91   Taixiang, W., Munro, A.J., Guanjian, L. "Chinese medical herbs for chemotherapy side effects in colorectal cancer patients". *Cochrane Database of Systematic Reviews* 2005, Issue 1. Art. No.: CD004540. DOI: 10.1002/14651858.CD004540.pub2.

of certain immune cells ("killer T-cells"), and also helps them reproduce. Interestingly, further tests showed that the drug did *not* enhance the ability of cancer cells to reproduce.[92] This is a good example of the selectivity of herbs between cancer cells and normal cells.

This research confirms what Chinese physicians have known for hundreds of years, that huang qi strengthens the immune system.

Reducing nausea

Chemotherapy can deplete the digestive qi of the body, which is why it causes nausea in many people. Nausea is one of the most common side effects on chemotherapy, and can be very debilitating. Many Chinese herbs have long been known to treat nausea, and there is growing evidence that Chinese herbs have a role in reducing nausea caused by chemotherapy.

A large trial, conducted by the Department of Clinical Oncology in the Prince of Wales Hospital, Hong Kong, investigated the use of Chinese herbs in treating the side effects of chemotherapy. One hundred and twenty patients were randomly assigned to two groups: one group were given a standard herbal formula for reducing nausea, while the other were given a non-therapeutic tea which tasted and smelt like the therapeutic herbs. The patients did not know which drink they were receiving. The study found that "the incidence of grade 2 nausea…was significantly reduced in the CHM [Chinese Herbal Medicine] group". In the group taking the false formula, 36 per cent suffered grade 2 nausea, while in the group taking the genuine formula, only 14.6 per cent suffered grade 2 nausea. The study

---

92   *The Journal of Immunology* (2008;181:7400).

concluded that Chinese herbal medicine "does have a significant impact on control of nausea".[93]

Maintaining kidney function

Some forms of chemotherapy, such as cisplatin, are toxic to the kidneys. A study was undertaken to see whether a certain herbal formula was effective in maintaining kidney function during the administration of cisplatin. Eighty-six patients receiving the drug were divided into two equal groups, one receiving the herbs, and one not. The patients received chemotherapy over four cycles, each of three weeks. In the group not receiving the herbs, significant changes were measured in the levels of blood urea nitrogen and creatine after completion of the treatment, indicating impaired kidney function. However, in the group receiving the herbs, no significant change was measured, indicating maintained kidney function.[94]

Getting through surgery

In Chinese medicine it is recognised that surgery can cause stagnation of blood, as well as depletion of qi. Often the surgery cuts a meridian, and blocks the flow of qi into the area which needs it most, the area where the cancer has developed. By supporting the qi, and helping move the blood, Chinese herbs are used to try and promote the healing process following the operation.

---

93   The trial was double blind, placebo, randomised and controlled. See Mok *et al. Annals of Oncology* (official journal of the European Society for Medical Oncology/ESMO), 2007 Apr;18(4):768–74. Epub 2007 Jan 17.

94   Mai Guofeng *et al.* "Clinical observation of Jian Pi Li Shi Ke Li in the prevention and treatment of renal damage caused by cisplatin". *New Drugs of Chinese Materia Medica and Clinical Pharmacology* 2000;11(3):136–7.

An investigation was carried out by the Breast Diseases Centre of the People's Hospital, Beijing Medical University, into the use of Chinese herbs for helping patients recover from breast cancer. Eighty postoperative patients were divided into two groups, one of which was given daily injections of a Chinese herbal formula for seven days. It was observed that the group receiving the formula showed a quicker return of haemoglobin to normal levels. It was also observed that "the wound healing time and postoperational complication in the treated group were less than those in the control group". The principal herbs used in the formula were ginseng (ren shen) and ophiopogon (mai men dong).[95] Ginseng is one of the most important Chinese herbs for strengthening the qi and blood, and is noted for its positive effects on the immune system in particular. Ophiopogon strengthens the yin, and generally strengthens the digestive system and the circulatory system.

Other side effects

A detailed discussion of the treatment of all side effects of radio- and chemotherapy with herbal medicine is well beyond the scope of this book. These include cardiotoxicity, liver toxicity, cystitis, ulcers and radiation pneumonitis (for a detailed discussion see chapter four of Li Peiwen, see Footnote 58).

SUMMARY

We have seen that strategies for the management of cancer with Chinese herbs have evolved over many centuries. The modern Chinese approach is to combine the wealth of knowledge

---

95   Liu, P. *et al.* Zhongguo Zhong Xi Yi Jie He Za Zhi. *Chinese Journal of Integrated Traditional and Western Medicine* 2000 May;20(5):328–9.

about herbs with the best of modern research. This research takes many forms. Pharmacological investigation has identified certain active compounds in certain herbs which exercise anti-cancer activity. Clinical trials have identified certain herbs and formulae which have helped fight certain cancers, and the quality of these trials is constantly improving. Some research is attempting to measure the benefits in terms of reduced side effects of treatment, and better quality of life.

Amidst the desire for high quality research, commendable though this is, it is important not to lose sight of the traditional Chinese approach, which seeks to design the best herbal formula for each individual. The therapeutic results of such an approach are, by their very nature, hard to measure, as every patient is given a unique formula. The biochemistry of a complex herbal formula is way beyond current levels of scientific understanding.

The Chinese approach is always to treat the person as a whole. It is important to support the person through unpleasant side effects, and to strengthen their body and mind wherever possible.

In addition to the complexity of the herbal intervention, we will find in the rest of this book that the Chinese approach involves many other complex interventions, which makes research even harder to undertake. The nature of modern research is to test one variable at a time, and keep the others constant. The physician of Chinese medicine, on the other hand, will seek to help the patient change many variables in their lives at once. To do anything less may even be considered unethical: the task of the physician is to do as much as possible to help the patient, in order to give them the best possible chance of fighting cancer, and improving their quality of life. In traditional Chinese medicine, herbs were never given in isolation from the other interventions explored in this book.

RESOURCES
Finding a good herbalist

The key to success with herbal medicine is in making an accurate diagnosis, and in selecting the correct herbs. A good herbalist will take a full case history, asking detailed questions about bodily functions, such as sleep, bowel movements, period cycle and emotions. They will make a careful examination of the patient's tongue and pulse. Based on this information, they will construct a herbal formula.

When talking to a potential herbalist, patients may wish to ask how long they have been in practice, and whether they have had any experience in working with cancer.

The regulation of herbal medicine varies widely throughout the West (a summary is given below). Where approved registers exist, patients are strongly advised to seek practitioners who are on such registers. Such registers will expect members to have received appropriate standards of training, and to abide by codes of ethics.

What kind of herbs to take

When selecting a potential herbalist, one should ask what form of herbs they use, as there are many ways in which herbs may be administered. The traditional Chinese method is decoction, which involves boiling the raw herbs in a pot for about 20 minutes. The knowledge that has been accumulated over centuries about how individual herbs work is based on using decoctions. If one uses a different method of taking herbs, there is no guarantee that the herb will work in the same way. Certain ingredients are extracted only by this method, and not by other methods. In the opinion of most Chinese doctors herbs should be taken in this form, at least in the short term while the cancer is active.

Herbs can also be given as concentrated powders. This is where the herb has been processed (usually in a factory) to make a powder. Sometimes this is done by boiling the herbs, then spraying the liquid onto starch grains. One of the drawbacks of this method is that some of the key compounds in the herb may be lost, especially the volatile oils. One may also lose the synergistic effect of boiling the herbs up together. On the plus side, powders are easy to take, and do not need to be boiled. When the patient is very fatigued, they may lack the energy or motivation to boil the herbs up. Powdered herbs are also significantly cheaper than raw herbs, if finance is an issue. This form of herb may be appropriate if the patient is taking herbs for extended periods, and is, for example, in remission, or in recovery.

One can put the powders into capsules if desired. This may be helpful if the patient is unable to drink the herbs, which sometimes happens if the patient has nausea. However, this means that the herbs have even less chance to work synergistically with each other. It also means that the dose is effectively much lower, as one can only take a small amount of powder in capsules, unless one is prepared to take huge numbers of capsules.

Herbs can also be prepared as tinctures. This is where the herb is soaked in alcohol for a period of time (usually several weeks at least). This method is very convenient, as the herbs are ready to take without any preparation. However, certain key ingredients in the herbs may not be extracted by this method, so the herb may not work in the right way. Preparing herbs in alcohol also makes them more heating, because alcohol has a heating effect. If patients are suffering from heat toxins, which they often are with cancer, using tinctures is not a good idea. Also, by altering the taste of the herbs, alcohol alters their energetic properties. As we shall see in the chapter on nutrition, the taste of things is very important for how they work. I do not recommend tinctures for those with cancer.

One can also take herbs as pre-prepared tablets, called "patent herbs" (the name patent herbs is misleading, they are not generally patented). However, because one has not designed the formula for the individual patient, it will probably be less effective. The dose is also much smaller than with a decoction. Patent herbs are not therefore generally used much in the early stages of cancer management. However, if patients are in remission, this is a cheap and convenient method of taking herbs over a long period of time.

In the United Kingdom, the Register of Chinese Herbal Medicine has set up an "Approved Suppliers Scheme". In order to become Approved Suppliers, companies who supply Chinese herbal products have to comply with certain standards. These standards include quality checks on herbs, appropriate training and care of staff, and not using endangered species. When choosing a herbalist, one may wish to ask whether they obtain all of their herbs from Approved Suppliers.[96]

The use of western herbs

I am sometimes asked why I use Chinese herbs rather than western herbs, given the ecological issues about transporting herbs from China. There are several reasons.

We have seen that Chinese herbs are selected according to their energetic nature. Over 2000 years, the properties of Chinese herbs have been extensively studied and documented, according to the Chinese energetic system. It has been established, for example, which herbs "subdue liver yang", which herbs "nourish lung qi", and which herbs "clear hot phlegm in the stomach". We do not have this kind of knowledge yet about western herbs. Although western herbs were used according to their energetic

---

96 For a full list of approved suppliers contact the RCHM via their website at www.rchm.co.uk.

properties historically, a different energetic system of classification was used. Western traditional medicine had four elements, rather then the five which the Chinese use. The organs were also conceived differently. This makes it very hard to fit western herbs into the Chinese way of working.

Another issue concerns the way herbs work with each other. It has been established in Chinese medicine which herbs work synergistically with each other. It has been established how herbs interact, and whether certain herbs prevent others working properly. It is therefore hard to drop the odd western herb into a Chinese formula, as we do not know how it will work with the other herbs in there.

Furthermore, as regards cancer formulae, there is very detailed clinical experience of using certain groups of herbs together in China. One cannot necessarily add new herbs to a formula and expect the same result.

Another issue is the method of preparation. We have seen that Chinese herbs are traditionally decocted. Western herbs, on the other hand, are more often made into tinctures, or infused (allowed to soak in hot water, like making tea). If one started to boil western herbs with Chinese herbs, they would not necessarily work in the usual way, as understood by western herbal medicine.

Having said all of the above, some writers are starting to try and classify western herbs according to Chinese energetic patterns, notably Jeremy Ross[97] and Peter Holmes.[98] This is an exciting and promising area, but it will take a very long time accurately to analyse even the most common few hundred western

97   Jeremy Ross (2003) *Combining Western Herbs and Chinese Medicine*. Bristol: Greenfields Press.

98   Peter Holmes (2000) *The Energetics of Western Herbs: Treatment Strategies Integrating Western and Oriental Herbal Medicine*. Boulder, CO: Snow Lotus Press.

herbs according to the Chinese classification system, and to work out how the herbs interact synergistically. Then one would have to develop this knowledge into a specialist area such as cancer. This could take several decades at least.

Registers of herbal medicine

If one is looking for a herbalist and an acupuncturist, it makes sense to see if one person can give both kinds of treatment. Most Chinese herbalists are also acupuncturists, but many acupuncturists are *not* Chinese herbalists. It therefore makes sense to look for a Chinese herbalist first, rather than an acupuncturist.

Some therapists are trained only to use patent herbs (tablets). Courses in patent herbs are usually only one year or less, as opposed to at least three years to become a full Chinese herbalist. One should check that a herbalist has done a full three-year training.

UNITED KINGDOM

It is recommended that patients consult a member of the Register of Chinese Herbal Medicine. The Register ensures that Chinese herbalists have received a full and proper training, of at least first degree level standard. The Register also sets a Code of Ethics, which all members must abide by.

UNITED STATES

There is much variation between States. Some states require herbalists to belong to registers, while others do not. One needs to discover the position in one's own state.

There is also a national register of practitioners, the National Certification Commission for Acupuncture & Oriental Medicine (NCCAOM). This organisation has a website, which allows people to search for a registered practitioner in their area: www. nccaom.org. Some states require practitioners to be certified with this body.

AUSTRALIA

There is a national register of Chinese herbalists: the Australian Acupuncture and Chinese Medicine Association (AACMA). This organisation has a website: www.acupuncture.org.au, which allows patients to find a practitioner in their area.

Chinese herbalists in Victoria must be registered with the Chinese Medicine Registration Board of Victoria: www.cmrb. vic.gov.au. This website also has a practitioner search facility.

CANADA

The position varies between provinces, with some regulating herbal mediicne, and others not doing so. The Chinese Medicine and Acupuncture Association of Canada has a website which allows one to find practitioners: www.cmaac.ca.

CHAPTER FIVE

Nourishing the Soul: The Chinese Approach to Nutrition

INTRODUCTION: THE CHINESE APPROACH TO A "BALANCED DIET"

The Chinese have known for over 2000 years that a good diet is crucial for health. When one has cancer, it becomes even more important, and this fact is increasingly backed up by modern scientific studies. Some foods contain chemicals which *inhibit* cancer growth, and other foods contain chemicals which *promote* cancer growth. The Chinese have identified many key foods which can be used in the fight against cancer, and modern research has confirmed and refined this knowledge.

If modern research has identified the foods which fight cancer, why do we need the Chinese approach? The key lies in the Chinese understanding of the *energetic* properties of food. Over the last two millennia, the Chinese have classified all foods according to whether they are hot or cold, dry or damp, toni-fying or clearing. They have also identified which foods treat which organs. This means that once a diagnosis has been made for a patient, they can select those foods which are suitable for their own energetic pattern. For example, a cold person should eat more warming foods, and a deficient person should eat more tonifying foods. Similarly, a person with a liver imbalance can ensure they choose foods which strengthen the liver, and a person with a kidney imbalance can select those foods which strengthen the kidneys. This is confirmed by research which shows that each particular organ, and each particular kind of body tissue, needs high levels of particular nutrients to thrive. For example, cervical tissue needs more vitamin C and folate than, say, gall bladder tissue, and a deficiency of those nutrients increases a woman's chances of cervical cancer.[99]

In the West, we often tend to identify certain foods as "good", and others as "bad". This classification changes over time, with the latest piece of research often overturning the previous one. Soya, for example, has been identified as helpful in fighting can-cer according to some research, but harmful according to other research. Some research claims to show that a vegan diet is best, but other research says that some animal products are beneficial. The basic Chinese position, on the other hand, is that a little of everything is good, and too much of any one thing is bad. One could summarise the approach as "moderation in all things". Foods are not usually "bad" in themselves, but *too much* of them can cause illness. In our society we tend to consume too much red meat, dairy, wheat, salt and sugar. These foods are not in-herently "bad"; indeed they can be positively beneficial for cer-tain people at certain times: problems only occur when there is over-consumption. Many people go to the extreme of rejecting

99   Blaylock, R. (2003) *Natural Strategies for Cancer Patients.* New York: Twin Streams, p.10.

"bad" foods entirely, which can, ironically, lead to other kinds of imbalances.

The Chinese emphasis on moderation and variety is backed up by our increasing understanding of the complexities of food. Whereas until fairly recently nutritional advice had been to ensure consumption of a few key vitamins and minerals, we are now finding that food contains thousands of compounds which have a profound physiological effect on our bodies. In order to ensure we get all the available compounds, it is necessary to consume a very wide variety of foods. For example, a group of chemicals called flavonoids, of which there are over 5000, are now being extensively analysed, and several dozen have been identified which have anti-cancer properties.[100] These key compounds are present in varying amounts, in varying foods. In order to get the complete range of the flavonoids, one needs to consume all varieties of vegetables and fruit.

We shall see in the section on the Five Elements that consuming balanced amounts of the five colours ensures one is getting a good range of nutrients. Again, this is being borne out by modern research, which shows that foods of certain colours contain certain key nutrients. For example, green foods contain compounds which help detoxify the liver. Yellow/orange foods contain high levels of beta carotene. Red foods often contain high levels of lycopene, which helps against prostate cancer.

Cooking methods

This is often an area of great controversy. Some nutritionists say that people with cancer should always consume a large amount of raw food, because cooking destroys some of the key nutrients found in food. The Chinese approach, however, is that raw food

---

100   ibid, p.257 (see Footnote 99).

has a very cooling effect, and is often not appropriate for those who have a diagnosis of *cold*. So how can we deal with this controversy?

We must first realise that there is a difference between the amount of nutrients *contained* in food, and the amount of those nutrients that one actually *absorbs*. While it is true that raw food contains very high levels of nutrients, those with a weak digestive system may not be able to absorb these nutrients. The nutrients in vegetables are locked inside thick cell walls, which weak digestive systems may not be able to break down. This is why the Chinese traditionally recommended methods to prepare food that would "warm" the food. This corresponds to making it more easily digestible, so that warmth and energy can be extracted by those with a weak "digestive fire". These methods included finely chopping food, grinding it down, mashing it up, lightly steaming it for a minute or two, or briefly stir frying it. These methods may slightly reduce the nutrient content, but this is more than compensated for by the increased absorption of nutrients.

The Chinese have long believed that it is also very important to chew one's food properly, thus breaking down cells walls and increasing nutrient release. It is also crucial to eat food in a relaxed, calm atmosphere. This allows the nervous system to switch into "relaxation" (parasympathetic) mode, helping maximise the amount of digestive enzymes produced, increasing blood flow to the gastrointestinal tract, and facilitating peristalsis. Unfortunately, many people opt for "fast food", and eat in less than calm surroundings.

Another option to be considered is juicing or blending food. We can think of this as a modern equivalent of grinding or mashing food. It breaks down the plant cells walls, allowing the nutrients to be released. In Chinese terms, this makes food warming, so is appropriate for people with cold conditions. Those who are very cold can add warming spices, such as ginger or cinnamon, to the mix. By releasing nutrients, juicing and blending makes food more tonifying. There is evidence that juicing and blending can be very helpful indeed for those with cancer, and I have seen people do very well on this method.

We can classify cooking methods according to how warming or cooling they are. These methods can be used to modify the energetic patterns of those eating them. In approximate order from the most cooling to the most warming, we can list these as:

- raw

- sprouted

- marinated

- juiced/blended

- fermented

- steamed

- boiled

- pressure cooked

- stir fried

- baked

- roasted

- grilled/barbequed

- deep fried.

Grilling and barbequing meat is not recommended for those with cancer, as it can produce large amounts of compounds called heterocyclic amines, which are carcinogenic.[101] It is not recommended to use microwave cookers, as these alter food enough to cause "structural, functional and immunological changes" in the body. Microwaves transform the amino acid L-proline into D-proline, a proven toxin to the nervous system, liver, and kidneys.[102]

In general, cooking methods that involve more cooking time, higher temperatures, higher pressure, and less water, impart more warming energy to food.[103]

Plants which take longer to grow are generally more warming (such as root vegetables), while those which grow quickly are generally more cooling (such as lettuce and cucumber). Using chemical fertilisers to make plants grow more quickly makes them more cooling. Food which is eaten cold is more cooling than food which is warmed up.

We shall examine the thermal properties of various foods below, in the Eight Principles section.

Food supplements

The issue of whether or not to take food supplements, and which ones to take, is controversial. The issue of supplements is beyond the scope of this book, and there are many other good sources which discuss this issue in detail.[104] One thing is clear, however: food supplements can never be a substitution for a good diet, for several reasons.

First, as mentioned above, we have only just begun to discover some of the huge amount of anti-cancer compounds in

---

101   ibid, p.23 (see Footnote 99).
102   Lubec, G. *et al. The Lancet* 1989 Dec 9;2(8676):1392–3.
103   Pitchford, P. (1993) *Healing With Whole Foods.* Pitchford, CA: North Atlantic Books.
104   ibid.

food. Large numbers of these compounds are not available as supplements. As more and more compounds are identified, one would have to take a huge amount of tablets to get all the required nutrients.

Food compounds often work synergistically together, enhancing each other's effectiveness: two plus two can often make ten. Sometimes certain compounds neutralise the negative effects of other compounds in a particular food, which makes it very hard to overdose on food. On the other hand, when supplements are taken, this balancing effect is lost, and one can more easily overdose.

It has been shown that certain synthetic forms of nutrients are at best useless, and at worse harmful. For example, vitamin C taken in the form of ascorbic acid can induce acidosis. This excess acid can prevent enzymes working properly, harming the digestive process, which is the last thing a person with cancer needs. Synthetic vitamins can also prevent absorption of other nutrients. For example, synthetic beta carotene can interfere with the absorption of another carotenoid, known as lutein.[105] Instead of nutrients working *synergistically* together, they can work *antagonistically* when taken as supplements.

Another problem is that synthetic vitamins often only contain one component, whereas natural forms contain a full range of components. For example, vitamin E is composed of eight different components, some of which have a strong anti-cancer effect. Some synthetic forms of vitamin E, however, have very little anti-cancer effect.[106]

Having said all of this, we would be no means rule out the use of supplements in those with cancer. We would merely advise that if one wishes to take supplements, it should be done under the guidance of a fully qualified and experienced nutritional

---

105   ibid, p.12.
106   ibid, p.12.

expert. We would also repeat that supplements must never be used to replace a high quality, varied diet, tailored according to the energetic presentation of the individual.

Eating with the seasons

Another key aspect of the Chinese approach is eating according to the seasons. The seasons are divided into five in Chinese medicine, each corresponding to an element, and therefore to a particular organ. One pays special attention to the element and organ of the current season.

In winter, for example, one looks after the kidneys, which dislike cold. One eats more warming, nourishing foods, and uses warming cooking methods, such as roasting and baking. In spring, on the other hand, one pays special attention to the liver. Spring is the time to cleanse the liver, and it is appropriate to use more cleansing, cooling foods, such as steamed green vegetables, or raw salad if appropriate. One tends to eat less at this time, perhaps undergoing moderate fasts if appropriate.

We shall look at this area in more detail below in the Five Elements section.

How to use this chapter

The first step is to obtain a good Chinese medicine diagnosis. This should be done by consulting a practitioner of Chinese medicine, as accurate self-diagnosis is not possible for the lay person. Information on finding a suitable practitioner of Chinese medicine is given in the resources sections of the acupuncture and herbal medicine chapters. When talking to potential practitioners, patients are advised to ask them whether they are happy to discuss their diagnosis, because not all practitioners will do that. Patients can also ask potential practitioners whether they will discuss diet; most of them will have studied Chinese nutrition as part of their training, and be happy to do so.

In order to get a diagnosis which helps you select the best foods for yourself, you will need a practitioner to have studied the *Eight Principles* model. All herbalists should have studied this model, as it essential for the practice of herbal medicine. However, some acupuncturists may not have studied the Eight Principles, and may only use the "Five Elements" model. The diagnosis they will give you will be of little value in helping you get the most from this chapter.

Once you have an accurate diagnosis, you will be able to make good use of this chapter, by selecting foods which are appropriate to your own pattern. Remember that your pattern may well change over time, so you need to check in with your practitioner from time to time to see how things are changing.

THE EIGHT PRINCIPLES

Once one has a Chinese medicine diagnosis, one can select foods according to the Eight Principles. For example, if one is predominantly cold, one consumes more warming foods. If one is predominantly deficient, one consumes more nourishing foods. It is important to review the diagnosis frequently, because if the treatment is effective, the presentation will change. One must therefore modify one's diet accordingly, as treatment progresses. I have seen many patients who had been put on a warming diet many months ago, and have now become *too* warm by not modifying their diet as they came into balance. In other words, they have overshot the centre, and gone to the opposite extreme.

It is also important to remember that most people will display a combination of several principles. They may have some signs of heat, and some signs of cold. People with a serious pathology such as cancer are advised to use foods of *moderate* thermal nature (cool and warm), rather than foods of an *extreme* thermal nature (cold and hot).

In this section we shall look at foods which treat six of the Eight Principles, namely:

- heat
- cold
- excess
- deficiency
- external
- internal.

Heat

We have seen that one of the main diagnostic factors involved in cancer is *heat toxins*. This involves an accumulation of waste material, due to the body losing its ability to break down toxins properly. The liver is usually involved in this pattern, as the main organ of detoxification.

One of the causes of this pattern can be the consumption of excessive amounts of hot foods. Particularly damaging are those substances which contain heat toxins, such as refined foods (including grains and sugar); processed foods; coffee; cigarettes; drugs (prescription or illegal). High levels of alcohol and red meat can also contribute to this pattern, although moderate amounts of these may be appropriate depending on the diagnosis.

Refined foods are imbalanced by their very nature. For example, white bread causes a very quick release of energy, then a sudden fall. In other words, it has a very high "glycaemic index" (GI), which is a measure of how quickly energy is released from a food. Whole grains, on the other hand, contain compounds which release energy slowly. Many compounds in whole foods have a moderating effect on other compounds, which make the food easier to process, and less likely to cause toxicity.

Whole foods also contain much higher levels of fibre, which is necessary for proper bowel movements. When the bowel does not move properly, constipation can follow. Chronic constipation can create high levels of toxicity in the gut, because toxins in the food will be re-absorbed. This situation can contribute to cancer in the colon.

Processed foods contain high levels of chemicals, such as preservatives, some of which are carcinogenic. These chemicals can be stored in the body, especially when the liver is too overloaded to break them down.

The Chinese have long classified red meat as hot in nature, and tonifying. We can understand this in terms of modern research, which shows that red meat can cause acidosis (a build up of acid in the body). This will prevent certain enzymes from functioning properly, harming bodily processes such as digestion and detoxification. Red meat also contains high levels of arachidonic acid, which can contribute to certain cancers.[107] In addition, red meat contains high levels of substances which have a high take up rate by cancer cells. These substances include the amino acids arginine and methionine, and iron. The iron in red meat can very easily create an excess level of free iron in the body, which is very easily utilised by cancer cells. On the other hand, the iron in vegetables is joined to other compounds, and only released as the body needs it. In Chinese medicine, the consumption of too many tonic foods, when one already has a

---

107   Blaylock, p.231 (see Footnote 99).

high level of toxicity, is known as "tonifying the pathogen". If a person has a high level of heat toxins, it is advisable to cut out red meat from the diet.

Alcohol is also classified as warming. It may be appropriate for cold patients in moderation, but is certainly not recommended for those with high levels of heat toxins.

Those people with strong signs of heat, especially signs of heat toxins, should avoid the heating foods just mentioned. They should also ensure they do not have too many warming foods (listed in the section below on cold). They should select more foods from the following table:

Cooling foods

Fruits	Vegetables	Grains/ legumes	Other foods	Herbs and spices
Apples	Tomatoes	Soya products	Sea vegetables	Red clover
Bananas	Lettuce			Marjoram
Citrus	Cucumber	Mung beans and sprouts	Spirulina	Nettles
Watermelon	Celery	Barley	Yogurt	Peppermint
Pears	Mushrooms	Alfalfa sprouts	Crab	Dandelion
	Radish		Clam	Chamomile
	Broccoli		Wheat grass	
	Cauliflower		Barley grass	
	Asparagus			
	Spinach			
	Aubergine/ eggplant			
	Sweetcorn			

Very warming cooking methods should be avoided, such as roasting and baking. Food should primarily be lightly steamed. Juicing and blending food is good for hot people. A small amount of raw food may be acceptable, as long as there are not strong signs of cold.

People who are predominantly hot may be drawn to consuming chilled foods and drinks. However, this is never advised by Chinese medicine. Chilled foods weaken the digestive qi, as energy is required to get the foods up to body temperature. Foods should be eaten at least at room temperature, preferably warm.

Chemotherapy can be a major source of heat toxins. These toxins put strain on the liver, which tries to break them down. Some of the cooling foods identified above have a particular role in clearing heat toxins, as modern research is confirming. For example, celery has traditionally been used to cleanse the liver. It has now been found to contain high levels of the bioflavonoid apigenin. This substance inhibits cancer by reducing the amount of a certain enzyme used by tumour cells.[108]

Broccoli has also been used traditionally to cool and cleanse the liver. It has been found to contain high levels of a certain bioflavonoid (called kaempferol), which has been shown to inhibit the binding of oestrogen to its receptor. This prevents the cancer cells utilising oestrogen, and is therefore very useful in cancers which "feed" on oestrogen, such as some breast cancers.[109]

We noted above that high levels of free iron can "feed" cancers. Many flavonoids have been shown to bind iron, only releasing it when it is needed by the body, and can thus play a role in preventing iron being used by cancer cells.[110] Broccoli is very helpful in this regard. Broccoli also contains high levels of

---

108   The enzyme is known as cyclo-oxygenase, or COX.
109   Blaylock, p.185 (see Footnote 99).
110   Op cit. p.187.

compounds called "isothiocyanates", which stimulate phase two liver detoxification.[111]

Asparagus is traditionally used to strengthen the kidneys. Recent research has suggested it may help protect the kidneys from chemotherapy induced toxicity.[112]

Cold

Cold often contributes to the formation of cancer. By slowing things down, it creates stagnation, and this stagnation can lead to the build up of pathogens such as phlegm and blood stagnation.

Over-consumption of chilled foods is one of the most common causes of cold pathologies. Ironically, many people struggle to eat salad straight from the fridge, thinking they are doing the healthy thing, but in reality making themselves too cold. Such people usually look very relieved when I advise them to cut down on salads, especially in wintertime. They usually feel much warmer very quickly. Even worse is ice cream, direct from the freezer. People who are predominantly cold should avoid food that is not heated, including raw foods. Juicing or blending makes food more warming, and may be acceptable in moderation. A cold person should add a warming herb such as ginger or cinnamon to the mix.

More foods from the table opposite should be selected by those who are predominantly cold.

Interestingly, one should avoid very hot foods and spices, such as chillies and pepper. These heat one up initially, but cause heat loss through sweating, which is why they are consumed in hot countries.

---

111   Op cit. p.189.
112   Blaylock, p.102 (see Footnote 99).

Warming foods

Vegetables	Grains/ legumes	Other foods	Herbs and spices	Animal products
Carrots	Oats	Sunflower seeds	Ginger	Trout
Parsnips	Spelt	Sesame seeds	Garlic	Salmon
Cabbage	Quinoa	Walnuts	Fennel	Chicken
Kale	Rice*	Pinenuts	Cumin	
Leeks	Corn*	Chestnuts	Cloves	
Onions	Rye*	Caraway seeds	Cinnamon	
	Aduki beans	Dates	Basil	
	Lentils	Cherries	Rosemary	

* These are thermally neutral foods, and are acceptable for hot and cold conditions.

More warming cooking methods should be used. Slowly cooked stews and soups are particularly beneficial. Pressure cooking also increases the warming effects of food.

Excess

As we saw in Chapter One, an excess pattern is a situation where a pathogen is present. Whereas most disease in ancient China was due to *deficiency*, such as a lack of essential nutrients, much disease in the modern West is due to *excess*. Generally, too much food is consumed, with particular excesses of fats, refined foods, and sugar. The primary focus in such cases is therefore to reduce the consumption of many types of food. Whereas dietary strategies in ancient China tended to focus on nourishing the patient, it is often more appropriate nowadays to focus on clearing toxins from the body. Thus, there is sometimes more of a need for raw food, juiced food, and fasting.

Two important pathogens which can contribute to the formation of cancer are *phlegm* and *blood stagnation*. In this section we shall look at the role of diet in tackling these pathogens.

PHLEGM

Phlegm arises when the digestive system fails to break food down fully. The undigested food is stored in the body as phlegm. There are two causes of phlegm, which often exist together. Firstly, if the digestive qi is weak, it is unable to digest food fully. This is a *deficiency* condition, and we will look at this in the deficiency section below. In these cases it is necessary to *tonify* the digestive qi.

The second cause of phlegm is the consumption of those foods which tend to cause phlegm by their nature, which is an excess situation. In this section we will outline those foods which are most likely to cause phlegm.

The weaker a person's digestive qi is, the more foods they will be unable to digest. Those with strong digestive qi will be able to break down most foods, whereas those with weak digestive qi will have problems digesting many kinds of foods. If a person is unable to break down a food fully it is said that they have a "sensitivity", an "intolerance", or an "allergy" to that food. These three conditions are listed here in ascending order of severity. A *sensitivity* is a fairly mild reaction, which is often barely noticeable in the short term. An *intolerance* is more severe, where consumption causes bloating or nausea. An *allergy* causes a severe and immediate reaction, such as inflammation or vomiting. In Chinese medicine, any food which causes these conditions is likely to lead to the build-up of phlegm, as the food will not be fully broken down.

If such foods are consumed over a long period, they can cause irritation of the lining of the gastrointestinal tract. This may lead eventually to conditions such as colitis. This, in turn, will further impair the body's ability to break down and absorb nutrients. This sets up a vicious circle, as the lack of nutrients further weakens the body, undermining its ability to absorb nutrients. This will create still more phlegm. Such a pattern is often seen in cases of colo-rectal cancers.

The "solution" proposed by many nutritionists is to cut those foods out of the diet which are causing the phlegm to accumulate. However, this is only tackling one half of the problem, and ignores the *deficiency* aspect. What often happens with such a strategy is that patients go on to develop further intolerances. Over time, they can end up on a very restrictive diet, which lacks many nutrients. It is therefore important to address the deficiency aspect, which we will discuss below.

Dairy products cause phlegm in many people who do not produce the enzyme lactase, which is necessary to break down the lactose in milk. Certain milk proteins are also hard to digest. Milk contains high levels of oestrogen, which is known to feed certain cancers, particularly some breast cancers. Intensively reared cows also contain high levels of antibiotics, which can adversely affect the immune system. This is the last thing a person with cancer needs.

Cow's milk is the hardest to digest, goat's and sheep's milk are sometimes better tolerated. Yogurt is the best form of dairy, as it is less phlegm forming. It is more easily absorbable as the bacteria have started the process of breaking down the compounds. The best form of dairy is therefore goat's and sheep yogurt.

Whether or not to use dairy products depends on the diagnosis: if there is a lot of phlegm, it is best to avoid it. If, on the other hand, the person is blood deficient, and does not have phlegm, some dairy may be beneficial, as it tonifies the blood. If the person is a vegetarian, they may obtain certain nutrients from dairy which they may otherwise lack. As we shall see below in the section on blood deficiency, according to Chinese medicine, animal products tonify the blood much more strongly than plant foods.

Wheat is another food which can contribute to the formation of phlegm. Some of the compounds in wheat are hard to break down. Unfortunately our culture relies heavily on wheat, and the problem is exacerbated by the fact that most of it is consumed in a refined form. With phlegm based cancers, it is advisable to replace wheat with other grains. Oats and barley are much better, as they have a drying quality, which can help to counteract phlegm.

Phlegm can also be produced by certain oils and fats, but the body does need some of these nutrients. We can utilise today's knowledge to select oils and fats which are most beneficial. The worst are "saturated fats", which contribute to the build up of cholesterol, which we can think of as a form of phlegm. These fats are found in high levels in red meat and butter, which have long been classified as phlegm forming foods.

Less harmful are polyunsaturated oils. However, these too can contribute to the formation of phlegm. Modern research has shown that these oils are chemically unstable, especially when heated. They easily oxidise, becoming rancid, and producing free radicals, which can be a significant contributory factor in some cancers. Such oils include safflower, sunflower, corn, peanut, soybean and canola. These oils are found in many ready meals and commercial products, such as cakes, crisps and pastries.

When using oils, it is preferable to use extra virgin olive oil, which is a mono-unsaturated oil. These oils are much more chemically stable than the polyunsaturated oils just mentioned. In the section on blood deficiency below, we shall see that flaxseed oil is a very good oil to use. Fats and oils do have a role in nourishing blood and yin, so it is important to consume them. However, we should select those which do not cause phlegm. When cooking with oils, one can add a pinch of turmeric. This contains curcumin, which has a protective effect against free radicals.

We can distinguish between hot phlegm and cold phlegm. Hot phlegm is yellow and sticky, and tends to occur in people who are generally hot. Cold phlegm is clear and runny, and tends to occur in people who are generally cold. Different foods are applicable for each kind of phlegm. If one is not sure whether the phlegm is hot or cold, choose foods from each category, as follows:

Foods which clear hot phlegm

Mung beans
Radish
Pears
Grapes
Sea vegetables
Carp
Dandelion

Foods which clear cold phlegm

Ginger
Leeks
Garlic
Cardamom
Cherries

Foods which can cause phlegm

Dairy products
Wheat
Meat
Alcohol
Fats/oils
Sugar
Bananas
Citrus fruits
Raw food

BLOOD STAGNATION

This is a major contributory factor to many cancers. We have also just discussed how certain foods can lead to the production of heat toxins. In turn, these can cause the liver to overwork, leading to liver qi stagnation, which in turn leads to blood stagnation.

If blood stagnation is present, one should consume more foods which help to invigorate the blood. These include olives and cherries, which have a sour taste, the taste associated with the liver (as we shall see in the Five Elements section below). Other foods which invigorate the blood include beetroot and buckwheat. All of these foods, and many others which have traditionally been use to invigorate blood, contain high levels of rutin. This is a bioflavonoid which has been identified as having anti-cancer properties. Rutin strengthens the blood vessels and promotes blood circulation to the hands and feet. In terms of Chinese medicine, we can think of it as promoting the smooth flow of blood.[113]

---

113   Blaylock, p.258 (see Footnote 99).

When a tumour grows its own blood vessels to supply itself, we call this "angiogenesis".[114] We can think of angiogenesis as a form of blood stagnation, as it interferes with the normal flow of blood. Soyabeans contain high levels of a certain bioflavonoid called genistein, which inhibits angiogenesis.

Other foods which are traditionally used to move blood stagnation include aubergine (egg plant), crab, papaya, and peaches. (The peach *kernel* is used as a herb to treat blood stagnation, and is discussed in the chapter on herbal medicine. It is, however, highly toxic and must only be prescribed by a fully qualified and experienced herbalist.)

Several culinary herbs are thought to have an anti-cancer effect, and can be added to food when cooking. These include include basil, saffron and turmeric.

Foods which invigorate the blood

Olives
Cherries
Buckwheat
Beetroot
Aubergine (egg plant)
Crab
Papaya
Peaches
Basil
Saffron
Turmeric

114   Blaylock, p.181–3 (see Footnote 99).

Deficiency

In Chapter One we looked at the "Four Deficiencies", each of which can contribute to the formation of cancer. In this section we shall identify which foods can be helpful in treating these patterns.

BLOOD DEFICIENCY

This is a deficiency of the *quality* of blood, rather than the *quantity*. We can think of blood deficiency as a lack of nutrients in the blood. This can either be due to problems with absorption, or to a lack of nutrients in the diet. Problems of absorption are due to deficiency of digestive qi, and this is discussed in the section on qi deficiency below. In this section, we will discuss foods which nourish the blood.

Although we tend to overeat in our society, many of the foods consumed have little nutritional value, so one often sees patients who are blood deficient. This may correspond with deficiencies in key nutrients, such as minerals, vitamins and amino-acids. A full range of nutrients is essential in maintaining the healthy functioning of cells, and in maintaining the immune system. If cells are undernourished, they are more likely to malfunction. If the immune system is weak, its ability to fight cancer is compromised.

Blood deficiency can lead to blood stagnation, like a river without enough water. There is a saying that "blood is the mother of qi, and qi is the commander of blood". When the blood is deficient, the qi tends to become deficient too. It is therefore essential to address blood deficiency when working with cancer. If the blood is not strengthened, the effectiveness of other interventions will be limited. Although acupuncture is effective at moving qi, *it cannot tonify the blood if inadequate nutrients are consumed*. Diet is therefore crucial in tonifying the blood.

One cannot help but notice that many vegetarians and vegans are blood deficient. This is because, according to Chinese medicine, animal products are the strongest foods to tonify blood. This is simply because animals contain blood, whereas plant foods do not. By consuming the blood of animals, we are nourishing our own blood. We can understand this from a modern perspective, as the cell structures and components of animal products are much closer to those of humans. Thus, they contain more of those substances we need. They also contain those substances in forms which are similar to those found in humans, and in similar proportions. Human protein structures are much closer to those found in animal products than they are to those found in plant products. This fact is particularly relevant to those with weak digestive systems, who find it hard to break down and absorb nutrients, and rebuild them in the form needed. One finds that those with weak digestive systems often do not do well on a vegetarian diet.

A vegan diet is particularly not recommended for those with blood deficiency. For example, it seems it is not possible to obtain vitamin B12 from a vegan diet. In the past, B12 was provided by the micro-organisms in food, but with today's sterile kitchens we do not get any B12 this way. B12 is essential for the production of red blood cells, and therefore of energy. It is also essential for the proper functioning of the immune system. Symptoms of deficiency include fatigue, apathy, memory loss, depression and paranoia. Interestingly, these symptoms correspond to aspects of blood deficiency in Chinese medicine.

Some have suggested that B12 is obtainable from certain plant products, however, the Vegetarian Society advises that:

> There has been considerable research into proposed plant sources of vitamin B12. Fermented soya products, seaweeds, and algae such as spirulina have all been suggested as containing

significant B12. However, the present consensus is that any B12 present in plant foods is likely to be unavailable to humans and so these foods should not be relied upon as safe sources. Many vegan foods are supplemented with B12. Vitamin B12 is necessary for the synthesis of red blood cells, the maintenance of the nervous system, and growth and development in children. Deficiency can cause anaemia. Vitamin B12 neuropathy, involving the degeneration of nerve fibres and irreversible neurological damage, can also occur… Researchers have suggested that supposed B12 supplements such as spirulina may in fact increase the risk of B12 deficiency disease, as the B12 analogues can compete with B12 and inhibit metabolism (in other words, compounds which are similar to B12 are absorbed instead of B12).[115]

The society recommends obtaining B12 either from dairy sources, or from vitamin supplements. Patients with phlegm should avoid too much dairy, so vegetarians should use vitamin supplements. However, vitamin supplements, for reasons discussed, are not considered as beneficial as natural, whole foods.

Red meat is one of the strongest blood tonics. It contains high levels of many key nutrients that we need. Some people intuitively feel the need for red meat at certain times, particularly around their menstruation, when blood is lost from the body. As we have said above, however, red meat does heat up the body, and can cause phlegm. Whether or not to use it depends on the diagnosis. In any case, moderation should be exercised in the consumption of red meat.

White meat tonifies the blood, but is less heating than red meat, and is preferable for those with heat conditions.

Traditionally, fish is seen as a much less potent blood tonic than meat. However, it does contain many tonifying compounds,

---

115   www.vegsoc.org/info/b12.html accessed 20 May 2009.

such as omega 3 oils. Those with heat conditions can consume fish with a thermally neutral nature, such as herring, carp, mackerel, and sardines. For those who need warming, trout and salmon can be used.

Dairy products have been discussed above in the "excess" section. They do tonify the blood, but can lead to the formation of phlegm. Yogurt from goats and sheep is preferable.

Legumes, such as beans, peas and lentils are blood tonics. In terms of western understanding, they contain much higher levels of protein than most plant products.

Many seeds, nuts and dried fruits are blood tonics. Particularly beneficial are sesame seeds, dates, figs and apricots.

Flaxseed oil has been identified as having potent anti-cancer properties: Dr Max Gerson found his cancer patients did very well on it.[116] Flaxseed contains high levels of omega 3 oils, which can be helpful in fighting cancer. It also contains high levels of lignans, which are converted by bacteria in the colon into two anti-cancer chemicals (enterolactone and enterodiol) which have shown anti-tumour effects against prostate, colon and breast cancer. One study from Finland showed that women with high levels of enterolactone had significantly lower levels of breast cancer than women with low levels.[117] Because this effect relies on bacteria in the colon, it is undermined if antibiotics are taken. One study found that premenopausal women who take antibiotics frequently are more likely to develop breast cancer.[118]

Lignan also acts to inhibit aromatase, which is suspected of contributing to certain cancers. Lignan is found in extra virgin olive oil, but is lost when the oil is processed. We can therefore recommend extra virgin olive oil as an excellent blood tonic.

---

116 Pitchford, p.126.
117 Blaylock, p.141 (see Footnote 99).
118 Blaylock, p.143 (see Footnote 99).

According to Chinese medicine, those with rich blood have a shining face, and Psalm 103 praises God for providing olive oil "to make man's face shine".

Foods which tonify the blood

Grains/ legumes	Fish/fowl	Vegetables	Nuts/seeds	Fruit
Oats	Chicken	Red cabbage	Sesame seeds	Red grapes
Rice	Octopus	Carrots	Dates	Cherries
	Squid	Fennel	Sunflower seeds	Plums
	Perch	Spinach		Apricots
	Eel			Blackberries
				Raspberries

QI DEFICIENCY

People with qi deficiency will tend to have low energy, and to feel cold. They may have chronic digestive problems, or tend to get ill frequently. In order to tonify the qi, one needs to use energising, warming, and drying foods and cooking methods. One should avoid too much raw food and cooling food.

Foods which tonify the qi

Grains/ legumes	Fish/fowl	Vegetables	Spices	Nuts/Seeds
Oats	Chicken	Carrots	Garlic	Hazelnuts
Millet	Trout	Fennel	Ginger	Walnuts
Corn	Salmon	Sweet potato	Coriander	Black sesame seeds
Rice		Leeks		
Lentils				

YIN DEFICIENCY

Yin is the cooling, moistening principle. If yin is deficient, the person will tend to be overheated and dry. This condition is commonly seen in menopause, when the yin declines. Chemotherapy and radiotherapy also deplete the yin: because they are very heating they tend to overheat the body, and to dry it up.

When yin is deficient, one should use more liquids in food preparation, such as soups and watery stews. One should avoid drying cooking methods, such as roasting or baking.

Foods which tonify yin are generally cooling and moistening, but tonifying too. Many of these are the same foods as listed above in the foods to clear heat. However, foods which are especially beneficial in cases of yin deficiency are as follows:

Foods which tonify yin

Beans	Fruit	Animal products	Vegetables	Grains
Mung beans	Grapes	Eggs	Spinach	Spelt
Kidney beans	Blackberries	Dairy (goat's/ sheep's yogurt best)	Tomatoes	Corn
Black beans	Raspberries		Sea vegetables	Rice
Soya products	Mulberries			
	Bananas			
	Apples			
	Pears			
	Citrus fruit			
	Strawberries			

Because these products tend to be cooling and moist, an excess of them may lead to cold and damp, so caution should be used.

YANG DEFICIENCY

Yang is the warming, energising principle. Yang deficient people will tend to be cold, tired, and poorly motivated.

Yang deficiency is basically an extension of qi deficiency, with more severe symptoms. All of the foods listed for qi deficiency are applicable to yang deficiency. With yang deficiency, even more warming cooking methods should be used, such as baking and roasting. More warming spices should be added to food, as listed in the table here.

Foods which tonify yang

All foods which tonify qi (see above)	Cherries
Beef	Peaches
Lamb	Leeks
Venison	Ginger
Walnuts	Fennel
Chestnuts	Cinnamon
Corn	Garlic
Raisins	

We have discussed cautions regarding red meat above. However, if the person has no signs of heat toxins, and marked yang deficiency, a small amount of red meat should be beneficial.

External

External illnesses comprise acute infections, such as colds and influenza. There are two aspects to treating external diseases. First, it is necessary to treat the acute illness itself. Second, once the acute stage has passed, it is necessary to strengthen the immune system. This is often necessary with cancer, because it is often a weakness in the immune system which has allowed the cancer to take hold. Certain immune cells are responsible for fighting cancer cells, and when the immune system is weak, cancer can thrive. Chemotherapy can severely weaken the immune system, because it kills the immune cells as well as the cancer cells.

We shall discuss the two aspects of treating external illness in turn.

CLEARING INFECTIONS

According to Chinese medicine, acute infections are classified into two types, which we shall look at in turn.

Wind heat invasions

These are characterised by a predominance of fevers, as opposed to chills. They may involve a sore throat. Any phlegm produced will be thick and sticky, and yellow or green. For these illnesses, one can drink herb teas which are *cooling* in nature, which include:

Peppermint
Yarrow
Elderflower.

These herbs are diaphoretics, which means they promote sweating, which releases the "pathogen". One can also use the foods listed above to clear hot phlegm.

Wind cold invasions

These are characterised by a predominance of chills, as opposed to fevers. They do *not* usually involve a sore throat. Any phlegm produced will be thin, copious and watery. For these kinds of illnesses, one can drink herb teas which are *warming* in nature, such as:

Fresh ginger
Cloves
Cinnamon
Garlic.

These herbs can be used in cooking, both to treat and to prevent infections, in those with compromised immune systems.

Herb mixtures such as this are included in mulled wine. Providing there are no contraindications to taking alcohol, such as liver problems or excess heat patterns, this can be a good way to take the herbs. This should be done in moderation of course, and one small glass will suffice. Alcohol has a dispersing nature, which helps to clear pathogens.

One can also use the foods listed above to clear cold phlegm.

NB: If any infection persists, one should consult a herbalist. These herbs are also not a substitute for orthodox medical advice, which should always be sought.

BUILDING IMMUNITY

In Chinese medicine, the immune system is governed by the lungs. It is also supported by the digestive system and the kidneys. In order to build up immunity, therefore, it is necessary to strengthen those three organs, particularly those ones which have been identified by a practitioner as weak. We will look at how food can help to do this in the section below on the Five Elements, which looks at foods for each organ in turn.

Internal

All illness which is not of the infectious type just discussed is classified as internal. Internal illness must be correctly diagnosed and treated, according to the Eight Principles and the Five Elements. We will not go into detail here, as this material is covered throughout this chapter.

THE FIVE ELEMENTS

As we saw in Chapter One, each element corresponds to a particular organ. Each element also corresponds to a particular taste, so foods with that taste can treat the relevant organ. For example, sour is the taste of Wood, and the sour taste treats the liver, the Wood organ.

If someone has either a particular craving or a particular aversion for that taste, it can indicate in imbalance in that organ. For example, if someone craves sweet foods, it indicates an imbalance in the digestive system. Earth governs the sweet taste and the digestive system.

The five tastes should be used in a balanced way, and one should consume all of the tastes regularly. Too much or too little of any taste will produce an imbalance.

The five tastes should be used with the seasons: each element, and therefore each taste, corresponds to a particular season. Different amounts of each of the tastes should be used at different times of the year, and according to the particular diagnosis of each individual.

Each taste has a specific therapeutic quality, which can be used to harmonise and strengthen the body. For example, the spicy taste moves stuck qi, and the sweet taste tonifies.

Each taste is also associated with the particular colour of that element, and foods with that colour can be used to strengthen the relevant organ. For example, green foods are used to treat the liver.

We will now look at each element in turn, and its associated organ. We will suggest key foods that can be used to treat the main pathologies for each organ.

Water: the kidneys

Water corresponds to winter. At this time of year one needs to conserve energy, and build up one's reserves. One should therefore not fast at this time. Rather, one should choose more of the nourishing, tonifying foods outlined in the Eight Principle section, which treat *deficiency* conditions.

The kidneys store the *essence*, and this should be protected and nourished during winter. As we explained in Chapter One, the essence is the body's reserve of energy. Essence is increased by the consumption of animal foods, such as chicken soup (boiled with the bones); royal jelly (made by bees); and to a lesser extent milk.

The kidneys dislike cold, so to strengthen them one should generally use foods and cooking methods which are warming.

The taste associated with the kidneys is *salty*. Many people in our culture consume too much salt, which weakens the kidneys. Refined salt should be replaced by good quality natural salts, such as rock salt or sea salt, which contain much higher levels of minerals. Sea vegetables give very good quality salt, and contain many minerals which are needed by the body.

Salt has the energetic quality of moving inwards, sinking and gathering, which is appropriate for winter, when we need to conserve our energy. The salty taste helps to break up lumps, which is very appropriate for those with cancer. Sea vegetables have long been used for this purpose in Chinese medicine.

The colour associated with water is black. Many dark foods nourish the kidneys, as we shall see in the lists below.

One should establish the correct diagnosis of any kidney pathologies before selecting foods. As we saw in Chapter One, the basic kidney pathologies are kidney yang deficiency (tendency to fatigue, and cold), and kidney yin deficiency (inability to relax, and tendency to overheat). If a person has *both* of these pathologies, we can say they have a deficiency of essence (essence can be defined as the sum of yin and yang). People in this category can choose foods from both the following lists, in proportion to the amount of kidney yang and yin deficiency.

Foods which strengthen kidney yang

Grains	Vegetables	Spices	Animal products	Other foods	Fruit
Buckwheat	Onions	Dried ginger	Chicken	Walnuts	Cherries
Oats	Leeks	Cloves	Trout	Black beans	Grapes
Millet	Radish		Salmon		
Roasted rice	Carrots	Fenugreek	Tuna		
	Parsnips	Fennel	Duck		
		Cinnamon			
		Garlic			

One can select foods from this category to make hearty winter soups and stews.

Most of these foods are quite thermally neutral and balanced. Although yin tonics are slightly cooling in order to nourish the yin, they are not too cooling, as this would injure the kidney yang.

Many, perhaps most, cases of cancer involve the kidneys. Often people have become exhausted over a long period, and used up their reserves, their kidney essence. This situation is often exacerbated by the conventional treatment received, which can have a very draining effect. It is therefore essential that these people build up their reserves again, and diet is one of the main ways to do this.

Foods which strengthen kidney yin

Grains	Vegetables	Animal products	Other foods	Fruits
Millet	Water chestnuts	Sardines	Mung beans	Pears
Barley	Potatoes	Crab	Kidney beans	Grapes
Rice		Dairy		Blackberries
	Sea vegetables	Eggs	Black sesame seeds	
	Cabbage	Duck		
	Asparagus	Octopus		
		Carp		
		Perch		

Wood: the liver

Wood is associated with spring. This is a time for renewal, for shedding the old and making way for the new. After the resting phase of winter, spring is the time for activity. As there is more energy all around us, we need to eat less, and to cut down our intake of heavy foods such as animal products. Spring is the time for cleansing and fasting, which rids the body of excess fats, which were appropriate during winter. Spring is the time to cleanse the liver, the wood organ. This is an essential aspect of treating many cancers, which usually involve a build-up of toxins.

The colour associated with wood is green, and it is appropriate to eat more green foods during spring. Many green foods have a cleansing action on the body. Sprouted foods may be beneficial at this time, although caution should be exercised as some people seem to react negatively to them.[119]

Food preparation becomes simpler in spring, with more raw or lightly cooked foods consumed. Less oil should be used, to allow the body to become lighter, and to rise with the spring energy.

The taste associated with wood is sour. Sour has the property of breaking up stagnation and excess. Vinegar has a sour taste, and one should use high quality products such as rice vinegar or cider vinegar, to help remove stagnation and toxins from the liver. Vinegar is a strong substance and should be used sparingly.

Foods which cool and detoxify the liver, and remove stagnation

Grains	Vegetables	Other foods	Fruits	Animal products
Wheatgrass	Celery	Mung beans	Lemon	Yogurt
Barleygrass	Cucumber	Rice/cider vinegar	Plum	
	Lettuce		Apples	
	Watercress			

The sour taste also has an *astringent* quality, which means it gathers and collects. The liver stores the blood, and sour products

---

119   Video: "The Gerson Therapy" (1992) Charlotte Gerson.

help to build the blood. Sour fruits and berries are beneficial, such as raspberries, blackberries and black grapes.

For a full discussion of foods to build the blood, see the "deficiency" part of the Eight Principles section above.

Liver qi stagnation can lead to blood stagnation. For a list of foods appropriate to this condition see above in the "Excess" section of the Eight Principles.

Liver qi stagnation can also lead to the accumulation of heat toxins. For a discussion of foods appropriate to this condition see the "Heat" section of the Eight Principles above.

Fire: the heart

The season of fire is summer. At this time one must be careful to keep the heart cool and moist, as it has a tendency to overheat. One therefore uses cooking methods which are cooling and moistening, such as lightly steaming or sautéing. As in spring, one eats less, and cuts down on heavy, fatty foods. One uses more light, cooling foods, such as salads, sprouts, watermelons, apples and pears.

The heart is said to dislike heat. The bitter taste benefits the heart as it clears heat and keeps the heart cool. Bitter has a clearing, downward bearing effect, and helps the body clear toxins through excretion (moderation should be exercised in order not to create too strong a laxative effect). Where the patient is deficient, the *clearing* effect of the bitter taste should be balanced by adding some sweet foods, which are *tonifying* (as we shall see below).

One of the most common heart pathologies is *heart yin deficiency*. This is where the heart has been overheated over a long period, and the yin has become exhausted in trying to keep the heart cool and moist. This condition is often caused by emotional problems, and is usually worsened by a diagnosis of cancer.

For this condition we need to consume foods which strengthen the yin, which are listed above in the "Deficiency" section. We should select a mixture of foods which are bitter and sweet: bitter to clear the heat, and sweet to tonify.

The other common heart pathology is *heart blood deficiency*. Like heart yin deficiency, this problem is often associated with emotional problems. The difference is that with heart *yin* deficiency there is overheating, but with heart *blood* deficiency there is not. To treat heart blood deficiency, one should select foods that nourish the blood, as listed in the "Deficiency" section above. Especially useful are chicken, red grapes, cherries, oats, goat's/sheep's milk, and short grain (glutinous) rice.

Earth: the digestion

The earth element governs the extra (that is, fifth) Chinese season of late summer. This is a time for harvesting and gathering, when the expansive outward energy of summer pauses, before starting to contract and move inwards in the autumn. Just as earth is associated with gathering and storing the crops, it is associated with gathering reserves for the body, ready for winter. The sweet taste of earth has the function of tonifying. However, by sweet we do not mean refined sugar, but the natural sweet taste of foods like root vegetables. These foods tend to have the colour of earth, which is yellow/orange. Refined sugar should be replaced by natural sweeteners, such as rice syrup, barley malt, molasses and dates.

Cooking methods are used which bring out sweetness, such as roasting and baking. Roasted root vegetables strengthen the earth organ, the digestive system. Many of the foods which tonify the digestive system are complex carbohydrates, which provide a slow, steady release of energy. If the digestive qi is weak, one should avoid all foods with cold properties, and ensure all food is warmed up.

Those with weak digestive qi should not eat large meals, as they will not digest them fully, and phlegm will be produced. Meals should be eaten frequently, in smaller amounts. It is very important to chew well, in order to break down food properly, and avoid phlegm. One should also eat in a calm, relaxed atmosphere, in order to help the process of digestion. Stress causes blood to flow away from the digestive system, thus impairing digestion.

Food which strengthen the digestive qi

Grains	Vegetables	Fruit	Nuts/ seeds	Spices	Animal products
Rice	Carrots	Sweet apples	Walnuts	Fennel	Chicken
Short grain (glutinous) rice	Sweet potatoes	Dates	Hazelnuts	Ginger	Duck
	Parsnips	Figs	Sesame seeds	Cardamon	Trout
Oats (especially porridge)	Pumpkins	Peaches		Nutmeg	Salmon
	Fennel	Raisins		Cinnamon	Tuna
Millet	Leeks	Sweet cherries		Vanilla	Butter (unless phlegm is present)
Polenta	Onions			Aniseed	
	Cabbage	Red grapes			

The main pathology of the digestive system is *digestive qi deficiency*. As we have seen in Chapter One, the digestive system makes qi for the whole body, and a deficiency in this organ will lead to general fatigue and weakness. This pathology is usually present in those with cancer.

In addition to the sweet taste, one should use moderately spicy foods and culinary herbs which stimulate the digestive system, as listed opposite.

When the digestive qi is weak, it can lead to the production of phlegm, which is one of the most common contributory factors to cancer. See the section on phlegm in the "Excess" section of the Eight Deficiencies above for dietary advice on avoiding phlegm.

Metal: the lungs

The metal season is autumn, which has a contracting, inward moving energy. There is a tendency towards stuckness at this time of year, both on physical and mental levels, so the *spicy/pungent* taste is used to counteract this, as it has the quality of *invigorating and moving.*

The spicy taste also stimulates the digestion to work better, so that it can break down the heavier foods which are consumed at this time of year: spicy aromatics stimulate the production of digestive enzymes. We begin to choose more foods which help to build our reserves for the coming winter, and these tend to be heavier. The spicy taste helps to prevent these heavier foods causing phlegm.

The spicy taste helps to clear pathogens, thereby warding off colds and flu, which often strike at this time of year as the cold weather sets in. The lungs govern the immune system in Chinese medicine. As we have seen, it is particularly important for those with cancer to keep the immune system strong, in order to fight the disease.

We looked at foods and spices to clear colds and flus in the "External" section of the Eight Principles above. In this section we shall look at foods to strengthen the underlying lung energy.

The colour of metal is white. One can see from the list below that many of the foods which boost the lungs are white.

Foods to strengthen the lungs and the "protective qi"

Grains	Vegetables	Animal foods	Spices
Oats	Radish	Tuna	Ginger
Millet	Daikon radish	Carp	Garlic
Roasted rice	Turnip	Duck	Thyme
Barley malt	Cabbage		Mustard
	Onions		
	Leeks		
	Scallions		
	Cauliflower		
	Mushrooms		

As we have said, it is also important to strengthen the digestion and the kidneys in order to boost the immune system. This is because the lung gets its qi from those organs.

SUMMARY

There are many books on nutrition and cancer, which list the best foods to consume for this disease. The beauty of the Chinese approach, however, is that each person can design the diet that is best suited to their particular pattern. A diagnosis should be obtained from a qualified practitioner of Chinese medicine, and once this is obtained one can use this chapter to choose foods which will help treat any imbalances identified. It is important to remember that the diagnosis will change over time, as treatment progresses, so a new diagnosis should be sought on a regular basis, preferably at least once a month.

The Chinese approach is dynamic, not static. One's diet should constantly be modified according to many factors, such as the time of year, how one is feeling, what stage of treatment one is at, and other factors that are changing. Selecting the best foods is a joy and an art, which is mastered over many months and years.

FURTHER READING

Kastner, J. (2004) *Chinese Nutritional Therapy*. New York, NY: Thieme.

Pitchford, P. (1993) *Healing with Whole Foods*. Berkeley, CA: North Atlantic Books.

CHAPTER SIX

Cultivating Qi

CHAPTER CONTENTS

Introduction • Qi Gong • Environmental factors • Conclusion •
Resources

INTRODUCTION

In this book we have looked in detail at many ways to enhance
our qi flow. We have seen that acupuncture, herbs, diet, and self-
cultivation can all be used to nourish qi. We can go further than
this and say that *everything we do, everything we think, and everything*
we are surrounded by, has a profound influence on the state of our qi.

Every time we undertake a physical activity, we influence
our flow of qi. If we move lightly and softly, with a sense of joy,
our qi will flow freely. If we move heavily and with tension, our
qi will *not* flow freely. Whenever there is hardness or tension
in the body, the flow of qi is restricted. This is because tension
creates *resistance* to the flow of qi through the meridians. When
the muscles are tense, the qi gets stuck, and transforms into heat.
This heat causes pain and inflammation, which is felt as stiff-
ness and muscle ache. When the qi is prevented from flowing
properly, it leaks out from the meridians, causing us to become
qi deficient.

In the modern world, many of us spend long hours in front of a computer screen. This tends to cause the qi to stagnate, especially in the shoulders, neck and head. It is therefore essential to balance this with some form of exercise to allow the qi to flow.

The environments in which we live and work also create qi stagnation. The way our homes and offices are laid out has a profound influence on the way our qi flows. In this chapter we shall see that we can structure our environments to maximise our qi flow.

Particularly when one has a serious illness such as cancer, one must examine all aspects of one's life in order to get well. Only by doing this can we truly talk of a holistic approach. In the search for health and wholeness, no stone should be left unturned.

The causes of cancer are many and varied, and usually several factors are involved. For each person it is important to identify which particular factors are involved in their pattern, so that they can be addressed. Some people need to focus on nutrition, whereas others may already have a good diet, but feel stuck in themselves. Others will feel the need to engage in physical activity, whereas others will feel more drawn to exploring the spirit. It is always a question of finding the right approach for each individual person. Each person must find the key that unlocks their own pattern of illness, and each person has a unique key.

All aspects of our lives must be in harmony in order for us to find true health. In this chapter we shall look at a few more ways in which we can cultivate our qi in order to promote this harmony. However, this book has by no means given an exhaustive list of activities which promote health. That list would be as long as human history itself.

QI GONG

Introduction

Qi Gong is a loose term, which can be translated as "qi exercises", or "qi training". Its purpose is to enhance the movement of qi through the acupuncture meridians. It does this by creating softness in the body, causing it to relax. When we practise Qi Gong often, it creates a habit of moving softly, and in a relaxed way. We use Qi Gong to overcome our habit of tension and hardness.

When there is hardness, the qi flow is blocked. This may cause accumulation of phlegm and stagnant blood, which can contribute to the formation of tumours. Qi Gong can help to improve qi flow, thereby helping to disperse phlegm and stagnant blood.

There are three elements of Qi Gong: harmonising the body, the breathing, and the mind. One must adopt the correct bodily posture to open the meridians. One must breath deeply and softly to enhance qi flow. Correct breathing strengthens the lungs, which are the organs of immunity in Chinese medicine. One must also calm the mind, as this helps the qi flow smoothly.

Most people do not realise they are in a state of tension for most of the time. This tension is there even when they are asleep, and feeds into dreams. One wakes feeling exhausted and unrefreshed. We veer between a state of hyperactivity and collapse, between extreme yang and extreme yin. Qi Gong allows us to find the middle ground of balance. It also allows us to switch more easily between the states of work and rest, between yang and yin.

Paradoxically, we get much more done if we are in a state of relaxation and softness. We need less sleep, and we work more productively. As Lao Tsu said, we achieve a great deal with no effort.

In many ways Qi Gong has a similar effect to acupuncture, by promoting qi flow. However, whereas acupuncture is used to treat certain acupoints, Qi Gong has a more general and widespread effect on the whole body. People often ask me which is better, Qi Gong or acupuncture. I usually reply that acupuncture is very effective at first, when the person is very ill and needs external help. However, over the long term it is best to practice Qi Gong, because that builds one's qi from the inside, and gives more permanent and lasting health benefits.

We can distinguish between two kinds of Qi Gong, external and internal. *External* Qi Gong refers to the transmission of qi by a therapist to a patient. The therapist will have developed very strong qi through many years' practise. They will place their hands on or near the patient, and "project" their own qi into the patient's body. We will discuss this practice more fully below.

Internal Qi Gong refers to exercises done by a person to maintain or improve their own health. These exercises are usually simple and repetitive. They are done slowly and calmly, often in time with the breathing. Qi Gong can also involve standing very still for periods of time, with the meridians "open", which allows the qi to flow unimpeded.

Some forms of Qi Gong exercise are used to maintain general health. Other forms have been developed specifically to address illness, and are referred to as "Medical Qi Gong". As we shall see, some forms of Medical Qi Gong have been developed specifically for people with cancer.

History of Qi Gong

The earliest mention of Qi Gong practice is thought to be in Lao Tsu's book, the *Tao Te Ching*, written several centuries BC. As we have just mentioned, Lao Tsu says that the sage achieves much with little effort. If one tries too hard, one creates tension, which actually blocks the flow of qi. We can think of Qi Gong as cultivating the habit of *not doing.* When we stop making such an effort, the qi flows naturally of its own accord. This is known in Chinese as "wu wei". Wu wei can be translated as "doing without effort", or "action through stillness". When applied to Qi Gong, it means allowing the qi to flow naturally by itself, rather than forcing it to move.

Lao Tsu also says that the way to health is to *concentrate on the qi and achieve softness.* Softness is an important aspect of Qi Gong, and distinguishes it from western style exercises. When the body is soft, the qi flows, but when the body is hard, the qi is blocked. A cancer tumour is, by definition, an area of hardness. This hardness is a reflection that the qi is not flowing freely, and is stagnating.

Another Chinese philosopher, Chuang Tsu, mentions "breathing down to the heels", which is another important aspect of Qi Gong. This sounds like a strange idea at first, as we think of breathing as done exclusively by the lungs. However, for the Chinese, "breathing" has a wider meaning of exchanging qi with the outside world. This qi exchange occurs across the *whole* of the body surface. In Chinese medicine, the skin is the "third lung", because it has the function of "breathing". In Qi Gong, one learns to "breathe" with the whole body, to draw qi in from the outside, right from the head to the feet.

There are specific exercises which draw qi in from the earth, through the soles of the feet. There are other exercises of visualising the qi entering the nose and flowing right down to the feet.

By the time of the Han dynasty, in the third century BC, there are many detailed references to Qi Gong in Chinese literature. After the first century AD, Buddhism came to China from India, and aspects of Qi Gong were incorporated into various religious systems, much of which were kept secret until the 20th century.

Many styles were practiced, usually within a tightly controlled family relationship, or "master–disciple" context. Some forms of Qi Gong developed into strange esoteric practices of internal alchemy, which claimed to bestow immortality on practitioners.

In modern China, Qi Gong is generally practised outside of any religious context, purely for health purposes. It is recognised by the Government, and taught in universities. A great deal of scientific research has been undertaken, demonstrating the health benefits of Qi Gong. Evidence has also been collected which shows that the qi emitted by Qi Gong experts is measurable as infrared electromagnetic radiation.

External Qi Gong

This is where a Qi Gong expert projects his own qi into the patient, in order to stimulate his qi. The therapist usually holds his hand near the sick part of the body, and sends qi into the patient. For those who have received such qi, it can produce a very powerful effect. It has been claimed that healing produced by this method is merely placebo, but scientific studies have been done whereby Qi Gong practitioners have transmitted their qi into cancer cells in test tubes, and slowed down their rate of growth. Qi has also been transmitted into animals with cancer, and had similar effects. An American study looked at this area, and said that "in vitro studies report the inhibitory effect of qi emission on cancer growth, and in vivo studies find that qigong-treated groups have significantly reduced tumor growth or longer survival among cancer-infected animals".[120]

---

120 Chen & Yeung (Department of Psychiatry, University of Medicine and Dentistry of New Jersey) *Integrated Cancer Therapies* 2002 Dec;1(4):345–70.

Several biochemical studies have investigated the effects of a form of external Qi Gong known as "Yan Xi Qi Gong" (abbreviated to YXQG) on cancer cells. One study on prostate cancer cells showed that YXQG altered the expression of certain cancer genes, slowing their growth, and inducing apoptosis (cell suicide). There was no negative effect on normal cells.[121] Another study showed similar effects on pancreatic cancer cells, with five minutes of YXQG inducing apoptosis in the cancer cells, without harming normal cells. The authors concluded that their findings "suggest that external Qi of Yan Xin Qi Gong may differentially regulate these survival pathways in cancer versus normal cells and exert cytotoxic effects preferentially on cancer cells, and that it could potentially be a valuable approach for therapy of pancreatic carcinomas".[122]

An American study was set up to compare the effects of genuine Qi Gong to sham Qi Gong. Tumour cells were injected into mice, who were divided into three groups, receiving genuine Qi Gong, sham Qi Gong, and no Qi Gong. The tumours in the mice of the genuine Qi Gong group grew significantly more slowly than the tumours in the other two groups.[123]

As with the other approaches outlined in this book, the effects of Qi Gong are hard to capture using conventional research methods. Qi Gong works to balance the whole person, rather than to remove isolated symptoms. The case study approach can allow us to see more clearly the overall effects of Qi Gong, and one such study was carried out in a Korean University. Eight sessions of external Qi Gong were given (on alternate days) to

---

121 *Molecular and Cellular Biochemistry* 2008 Mar;310(1–2):227–34. Epub 2007 Dec 16.

122 *International Journal of Biochemistry and Cell Biology* 2006;38(12):2102–13. Epub 2006 Jun 27.

123 Chen *et al.* (University of Medicine and Dentistry of New Jersey – Robert Wood Johnson – Medical School, Newark, NJ, USA) *Journal of Alternative and Complementary Medicine* 2002 Oct;8(5):615–21.

a 35-year-old man with advanced cancer (Stage IV), involving metastases to the stomach, lung and bone. The man was disabled and required special assistance. The study reported that:

> A visual analogue scale (VAS) was used to assess the patient's self-reported symptoms of cancer over the intervention and follow-up periods. Following treatment, VAS scores' analysis revealed beneficial effects on pain, vomiting, dyspnoea [breathing problems], fatigue, anorexia, insomnia, daily activity and psychological calmness. These improvements were maintained over the two-week follow-up phase. After the first Qi therapy session, the patient discontinued medication and could sit by himself; after the fourth session, the patient was able to walk and use the toilet without assistance.[124]

Of course, there are limitations to the case study approach. It does, however, capture something of the profound and far reaching changes that Qi Gong can bring to people's lives.

Internal Qi Gong

This consists of certain exercises designed to stimulate qi in the meridians. Although there are many hundreds of forms, there are some basic principles shared by all:

- *Allow the mind to relax and let go:* this will take time, and must not be forced, as this will be counterproductive.

- *Allow the mind to guide the qi, and the qi to guide the mind:* the two should work in harmony, neither over-dominating.

- *Softness and emptiness in the upper body, strength and fullness in the lower body:* this is the opposite of how most people

---

124   Lee *et al. European Journal of Cancer Care* 2005 Dec;14(5):457–62.

exist. We tend to be tense in the head and neck, and weak in the lower body.

- *Moderation:* one must not over-exert, as this creates tension and weakness. In our culture we want results now, but the body has its own pace of healing, and trying to go too fast is counterproductive.

- *Recuperation:* after a session it is very important to allow oneself to relax for a while, especially if one is very ill.

- *Master the basics before moving to the complex:* again, we want to move too fast. If one does not embody the basic principles first, such as softness, advanced exercises will only create tension.

- *Practice regularly and steadily:* a little every day is best.

- *Do not practice when tense:* the qi will not flow.

- *Do not worry about unusual sensations:* these may include twitching, heat, cold, or itching, which are a normal part of practice.

One of the most popular forms of Qi Gong is the Ba Dua Jin, "Eight Strands of Gold Brocade". Each posture enhances qi flow in certain acupuncture meridians, and the whole sequence works all 12 primary meridians. This form can be done in about 20 minutes. When one has completed the form, one holds one's hands on a point below the navel called "Sea of Qi", in order to gather the qi there. The exercises are done slowly, in time with the breathing, keeping the body soft and relaxed, to promote the flow of qi.

It has long been known in China that the regular practice of Qi Gong tends to bring many health benefits, such as stronger immunity, calmness, increased fitness and improved energy levels. Much research which is now being done backs up these claims.

One study conducted by a Swedish University showed various psychological benefits from doing Qi Gong, including reduced anxiety and improved mood. Interestingly, the study showed that doing Qi Gong for 30 minutes was just as effective as doing it for 60 minutes, which is good news for those with busy lives.[125]

One fascinating study by the Centre for Immunology, in the University of Texas, looked at the effects of Qi Gong on the expression of genes. The genetic profiles of a group of Qi Gong practitioners were compared to that of a control group, who did not practice Qi Gong or any similar exercises. Immune cells (neutrophils) were extracted from the blood, and examined for genetic expression (in other words, for the activity of the genes). It was found that the cells of the Qi Gong practitioners displayed enhanced immune function, as well as enhanced ability to reduce inflammation. The cells also lived longer, and displayed an enhanced capacity for phagocytosis (the destruction of invading cells). The authors concluded that,

> our pilot study provides the first evidence that Qi Gong practice may exert transcriptional regulation at a genomic level. New approaches are needed to study how genes are regulated by elements associated with human uniqueness, such as consciousness, cognition, and spirituality.

This study has profound implications for cancer patients, whose immune system is often compromised.[126]

One Korean study attempted to measure the long-term benefits of Qi Gong, using 768 people who had practiced it for at least ten years. Subjects reported the following benefits of practicing Qi Gong:

---

125 Johansson *et al. American Journal of Chinese Medicine* 2008;36(3):449–58.
126 Li, Q. Z. *et al. Journal of Alternative and Complementary Medicine* 2005 Feb;11(1):29–39.

- general improvements in perceived physical health: 67 per cent

- improvements in perceived psychological health: 40 per cent

- reduced pain: 43 per cent

- reduced fatigue: 22 per cent

- reduced insomnia: 9 per cent

- increased resistance to the common cold: 60 per cent.[127]

Wound healing was also surveyed in 332 of the subjects, and of these:

- 84 per cent reported improvement in recovery time

- 67 per cent reported reduced inflammation

- 50 per cent reported improvements to scar tissue.

Some forms of Qi Gong are suitable for those who are very ill and unable to move much. These can be done sitting, or even lying down. As long as the meridians are open, and the body is soft, the qi flow will be enhanced.

Medical Qi Gong

This refers to systems which have been developed specifically for medical conditions. Medical Qi Gong is very commonly used in Chinese hospitals, for a wide variety of complaints. Certain forms have been developed specifically for those with cancer, and research is increasingly confirming the benefits. A meta analysis of over 50 trials on Medical Qi Gong for cancer was

---

127   Lee *et al. American Journal of Chinese Medicine* 2003;31(5):809–15.

conducted by the Department of Psychiatry of the University of Medicine and Dentistry, New Jersey, USA. They found that many of the trials showed evidence for Qi Gong increasing life expectancy.[128]

The Faculty of Medicine in the University of Sydney, Australia, conducted a study of the benefits of Qi Gong to people with cancer. They randomly assigned a group of 30 patients with various cancers into two groups, those who practiced Qi Gong for eight weeks, and those who did not. The researchers found that those who did the Qi Gong scored higher on the QOL (Quality of Life) Index, and also reported fewer side effects of conventional treatment. In addition, the patients practicing Qi Gong were found to have lower levels of inflammation generally, as measured by blood levels of a key biomarker (c-reactive protein).[129]

Chemotherapy kills normal blood cells, as well as cancer cells. A paper was published in an American journal on a trial examining whether Qi Gong could help this problem. A total of 77 patients undergoing chemotherapy for breast cancer were assigned to two groups, one of which undertook a form of Qi Gong known as Chan Chuang. After they had completed 21 days of Qi Gong, the patients in that group were found to have significantly higher counts of white blood cells, haemoglobin, and platelets. This would strongly suggest that Qi Gong may help boost immunity and general energy levels.[130]

Two Korean studies also suggest that Qi Gong improves immune function. One study found that after only one training session, the functioning of neutrophils (immune cells) was

---

128   Chen and Yeung (Department of Psychiatry, University of Medicine and Dentistry of New Jersey) *Integrative Cancer Therapies* 2002 Dec;1(4):345–70.

129   Oh *et al. American Journal of Chinese Medicine* 2008;36(3):459–72.

130   Yeh *et al. Cancer Nursing* 2006 Mar–Apr;29(2):149–55.

significantly enhanced. The authors concluded that "qi training may increase the resistance of trained individuals against common infection and inflammation".[131] In another study, a group performing Qi Gong was compared to a group performing "sham Qi Gong" exercises, where no attempt was made to move the qi. The Qi Gong group showed significantly higher increases in certain immune cells, and the authors concluded that "a single Qigong intervention can increase the monocyte and lymphocyte numbers".[132]

The Department of Psychobiology and Methodology of the University of Malaga, Spain, also conducted an experiment to observe the effects of Qi Gong on the immune system. A group of 29 subjects, who had not practiced Qi Gong before, was assigned to two groups, one of which practiced Qi Gong for 30 minutes per day for one month. At the end of the month, "significant immunological changes occurred between the experimental and control groups".[133]

One type of Medical Qi Gong practice of particular interest is "Guo Lin Qi Gong", named after its founder, a woman named Guo Lin (1906–1984). This style involves walking in a certain way, which is designed to free the qi in the body. In 1949 Guo Lin was diagnosed with uterine cancer and had surgery to remove it. In 1960 she had a recurrence and found it had spread to her bladder. Another operation was done to remove the cancerous portion of the bladder, but she relapsed again and was given only a few months to live. Not willing to give up her fight, she recalled the Qi Gong her grandfather had taught her as a child. She researched and practised, but did not feel much

131   Lee *et al. Journal of Alternative and Complementary Medicine* 2004 Aug;10(4):681–3.

132   Lee *et al. American Journal of Chinese Medicine* 2003;31(2):327–35.

133   Manzaneque, J. M. *Medical Science Monitor* 2004 Jun;10(6):CR264–70. Epub 2004 Jun 1.

benefit. So, she did more research into ancient writings, and then developed her own practice schedule for two hours everyday. After six months her cancer had subsided.

Based on her own experience, she believed that her style of Qi Gong could help others in their fight against cancer and other serious diseases. In 1970 she began giving lessons in "New Qi Gong Therapy". This combined movement Qi Gong with "quiet" Qi Gong, in which the person learns to allow the mind to let go of any negative thoughts and emotions. This helps to induce a state of calmness and relaxation. As we have seen, one's state of mind has a profound influence on qi flow: when the mind is relaxed, the qi flows smoothly. On the other hand, mental tension will produce physical tension, and block qi flow.

By 1977 Guo Lin had achieved many positive results, with many of her students testifying that their cancers had been put into remission or even gone. She became something of a celebrity in China, and her classes grew to several hundred students every day. She taught all over China until her death in 1984, aged 78, 24 years after she was supposed to have died.

Guo Lin's work fed into the network of Cancer Recovery Clubs which now exist in China. Several hundred thousand people have been through these clubs. Guo Lin placed great emphasis on the need for support, particularly from the family. Also, by practising in large groups, mutual support is generated. When one person makes good progress, other students are given confidence in the method, and encouraged in their own efforts. Guo Lin knew that a positive mental outlook is crucial in the fight against cancer. Her legacy is worthy of close attention in the West, where we could learn to pay more attention to the need for supporting therapies.

Healing Sounds Qi Gong

There are many different forms of this practice, based on the principle that sound vibration can harmonise specific parts of the body. Each organ is thought to vibrate at a certain frequency, and this can be enhanced by making the appropriate sound. One breathes in softly, then as one exhales, one makes the sound softly, with no tension. As we have seen, softness is essential for the qi to flow. One can focus on that part of the body being harmonised. The following is one kind of system commonly used, known as the "Eight Healing Sounds":

AAH: tonifies the lungs. This sound is made quietly. It helps the lungs take in the new and expel the old, as well as supporting the immune system.

HA: tonifies the heart. This sound is quiet and without tone. This sound regulates the yin and yang of the heart, and also clears heat.

HENG: tonifies the kidneys. This sound is short and sharp. It creates a strong downward movement of Qi, to fill the kidneys and nourish the essence.

HU: tonifies the stomach. This is a long droning sound.

MER: tonifies the digestive system. This sound is strong and resonant, and clears damp from the body.

SHHHHU: tonfies and soothes the liver. This sound is smooth and soft. It clears heat from the body, calms the mind, and helps the qi sink.

YEEE: this opens up all 12 primary meridians. One makes a clear and long tone. The vibration should reach the head and toes, and enter the brain and kidneys.

HONG: this further opens the meridians. One creates a

long, strong vibration through the entire body, opening all the meridians, and connecting them to the earth's Qi. The sound is a low guttural rumbling, extending from the centre to the extremities.

To gain maximum benefits, these sounds are practised along with a series of movements, but they can also be done by themselves. As with all Qi Gong, one should find a qualified and experienced teacher.

Another system is known as the "six character method" (liu zi jue). This is a similar idea, with a particular sound corresponding to each of the five elements (there are two sounds for fire). A Japanese experiment set out to test the effects of the sounds on pain, based on the Chinese medicine theory of the "control cycle". According to this theory, each element is controlled by another element. A pain was produced in subjects by pressing a certain acupoint. The pain was relieved by touching another acupoint and making the correct sound (according to the five elements control theory). However, if the sound of the wrong element was made, the pain actually increased.

The same team conducted another experiment to test how the sounds changed the electrical activity of acupoints. As we mentioned in the chapter on acupuncture, if an organ is out of balance, the electrical current will usually be abnormal in the corresponding acupoint. A person was tested who had an abnormally high electrical charge in a bladder point (8 milliamps instead of 1). Chanting the correct sound caused the charge to drop towards a more normal level (2.6 on the left and 5.2 on the right).[134]

The team also conducted another experiment to test the power of sound. Using a metronome to emit regular clicks, they

---

134 Manaka, Y. (1995) *Chasing the Dragon's Tail*. Philadelphia, PA: W.B. Saunders, p.97–98.

tested the frequency that reduced pain in each of the acupuncture channels. For each acupuncture channel, it was found that there was a certain consistent frequency which relieved pain (the frequencies for each channel varied from 104 to 176 beats per minute). A range of people were then treated for pain, and it was found that the treatments were enhanced when the metronome was set at the frequency of the channel being treated. No enhancement was observed when other frequencies were used.[135]

These experiments demonstrate the profound influence that sound has on the flow of qi. Conversely, negative sounds have a bad influence on qi. Loud, hard, heavy, thumping music will tend to disrupt the qi, and leave one feeling tense. It is not hard to see that much modern music can have a very negative effect, especially on young people, whose qi is not fully developed. From the Chinese perspective, heavy metal music and night clubs are bad news. They destroy a sense of peace, and create tension. This distorts one's normal rational perspective, and leaves one feeling the need of something to correct the imbalance. Thus one is drawn to take drugs and excessive alcohol, as one seeks some kind of "rebalance". Some may also crave sex in an attempt to release tension and gain a sense of peace. The combination of "sex, drugs and rock and roll" is ultimately a very dangerous one, as the lifestyles of many famous people have shown. It is the direct opposite of what the sages were trying to cultivate.

Visualisation Qi Gong

There is a saying that "qi follows the mind". If we use our mind to visualise the qi flowing, then the qi will indeed flow more strongly.

---

135   Manaka, p.72 (see Footnote 134).

One such exercise involves imagining a golden ball of light above one's head. The light slowly enters the top of the head, then gradually fills the whole body, down to the tips of the toes. Normally one stands or sits with eyes closed, while the teacher talks one through the exercise. On completion of the exercise, one feels very light, energised, and relaxed. Often one will feel tingling throughout the body, or a sensation of movement within.

Another exercise uses the five element colour–organ correspondences. Each colour can be used to strengthen the relevant organ. One visualises breathing in, and taking the qi to each organ in turn. The organ is seen in its appropriate colour, shining brightly. This exercise enhances the vibrational pattern of each organ in turn.

Another experiment by the Japanese team mentioned above was conducted into the effects of placing colours on the acupoints. A pressure pain was produced by pressing a certain acupoint. If the correct colour was marked on a certain other acupoint, the pain reduced. If, however, the wrong colour was applied, the pain returned.[136]

Summary

There are many forms of Qi Gong, and different forms suit different people. Some forms are more energising, while others are more relaxing. It is important to establish a regular daily routine, and to try not to miss a day's practice. One should aim for a little every day, and not over-exercise. Too much training in the early stages can leave one depleted. The most important thing is to find a well qualified and experienced instructor, who will guide you through the whole process. The practice of Qi Gong is a very

---

136   Manaka, p.92 (see Footnote 134).

important part of the fight against cancer, as it has a profound influence on the mind, and on the flow of qi in the body.

ENVIRONMENTAL FACTORS

Introduction

Man is intimately connected with his surroundings. According to Chinese thought, the human person is a microcosm of the whole universe. The flows of energy in the cosmos are mirrored by the flows of energy inside of us. We are not isolated units, but are deeply embedded in our environment. We are constantly exchanging qi with the rest of creation. We absorb qi from our environment, and are therefore deeply influenced by all that goes on there. Whenever the energy flow is disturbed around us, it will have an impact on our internal qi flow, and tend to make us unwell. If, on the other hand, we are able to surround ourselves with good qi, we will tend to feel well.

Similarly, when we breathe out our qi, we influence all around us. We are intimately connected with the other people around us, whether we like it or not. We each have a responsibility to cultivate our own qi, in order positively to influence other people.

From the most ancient times man has known that certain places felt good, and certain places did not. In the West the art of geomancy developed, which explored the influence of natural phenomena such as the "lie of the land", and watercourses. It also recognised that there were certain stress lines in the earth which could create health problems. We can today think of such lines as areas of electromagnetic disturbance.

One European tradition placed an ants' nest in the site of a prospective bedroom. If the ants thrived, the area was not used, but if the ants left, the area was deemed suitable. Ants thrive on areas of geopathic stress, which is the opposite to humans. Cats also thrive in such areas, whereas dogs do not.

In 1929 a German aristocrat called Gustav Freiherr von Pohl conducted an experiment in the town of Vilbisburg. He dowsed the town for negative energies caused by underground watercourses and earth stress lines. Each day he was accompanied by a policeman to ensure he did not speak to anyone. On completion of his study, his map of harmful areas was compared to a list of the 42 cancer patients in the town. It was found that all the patients lived in the areas of stress. The experiment was repeated in other towns with similar results.

Those with a serious illness such as cancer should take into account areas of electric disturbance, which can disrupt the normal flow of qi. Acupoints are areas of tiny electrical activity (around one milliamp), which can be disturbed by large electromagnetic fields. It is well known that electromagnetic energy fields disrupt nearby electrical currents.

Several studies have linked areas of electrical activity with certain cancers. A Japanese study into 312 children with leukaemia found that children living near electromagnetic fields were more likely to develop leukaemia than other children.[137] Several studies into mobile phones have showed that their long-term use is associated with an increased risk of brain tumours.[138] Young children are particularly at risk from electromagnetic disturbance, because their qi systems are not yet fully developed. Those with cancer should be especially aware of electromagnetic disturbances, which can be measured with the appropriate equipment.

In our times, ecological problems are forcing us to remember the importance of the environment for our well-being. If we look after the planet, it will look after us. If we neglect it, we will pay the price. Chinese medicine is essentially an ecological

---

137   Kabuto *et al. International Journal of Cancer* 2006 Aug 1;119(3):643–50.

138   Hardell *et al. Internationl Journal of Oncology* 2008 May;32(5):1097–103.

system of medicine, showing us that we can only be healthy if the planet is healthy. If we live out of harmony with nature, nature will become unable to sustain us. We can note the irony that as China industrialises, it is seeing many kinds of cancers rise rapidly towards western levels.

Feng Shui

In China the art of "finding one's place" was developed into a highly sophisticated system known as Feng Shui, which literally means "wind and water". It was recognised that good quality wind, in other words air, is essential for health. The air should not be too damp, or too dry. One should not live in a very exposed location, such as top of a hill, as this is unsheltered. As well as being at risk from the elements, such a location is more prone to energetic disturbances.

Neither should one live in too sheltered a location, such as in a deep valley, as this can create stagnation. Damp tends to gather in such places, and the qi cannot flow well. This tends to create a feeling of heaviness and stuckness.

If you were to analyse the area where you live from the perspective of Feng Shui, you would probably notice that the more affluent houses are sited in the most favourable locations, whereas the poorer houses have had to settle for the less favourable ones. Much of Feng Shui is instinctive: some places just have a better *feel* than others.

Similarly, we must also live in a suitable relationship to the water around us. On a basic level, the quality of drinking water has a great impact on our health. We can think of this in terms of cleanliness and mineral content. But we can also think of this in terms of the *vitality* of the water. The qi of spring water gives more vitality than the qi of stagnant water. Nowadays we just have to take what come through the pipes in our homes, although we can at least fit a filter. Bottled water has its own problems, in terms of negative environmental impact, and plastics leaching into the water.

Water can also create problems if the house is wrongly sited in relation to it. As we shall see below, water at the back of the house creates energy disturbances. Underground water also disturbs energy flows.

The art of Feng Shui was developed into a much broader practice than just looking at the air and water around us. It became the art of examining the movement of energy around us, and our interaction with that energy. When this movement is harmonious, we feel well. When this movement is disharmonious, we feel ill. The ancient Chinese explored the factors which created harmonious living spaces, and learnt how to choose those places which enhanced one's energy. Over time a detailed system was developed which recognised the "nine aspects" of environmental harmony, which were:

- History

- Philosophy

- Electromagnetic forces

- Cosmic energy

- Location

- Shapes

- Internal arrangements

- Timing

- The human dimension.

When any of these aspects are out of balance, we can feel tired, on edge, and restless. When each of these aspects is in harmony, one can create living spaces which feel peaceful, yet energising.

We all know that certain places just feel good, and others just feel bad. Feng Shui is the attempt to explore what makes for harmonious energy, and to enhance this energy so that we can live a harmonious life.

Feng Shui is often presented in the West as little more than a kind of interior design. In reality it is a highly complex and evolved art, which examines every facet of man's relationship with his surroundings. In order to master each of the nine aspects mentioned, they must be studied over many years. One should therefore always consult an expert before making changes (see "Resources" section below). This chapter can do no more than mention a few aspects about how Feng Shui works, and certainly does not allow one to implement its complex principles.

The Five Animals

We have explored the Five Elements in previous chapters, and seen how they should always be in balance with each other. No element should be too dominant, or too weak. For each of the nine aspects of harmony, the Five Elements should be balanced. In Feng Shui, the Five Elements are symbolised by five animals, as follows:

Water: tortoise

Wood: dragon

Fire: phoenix

Earth: snake

Metal: tiger

For a space to be harmonious, the five animals must be in harmony with each other. Each animal has a specific place, as follows:

Let us take a look at each animal in turn.

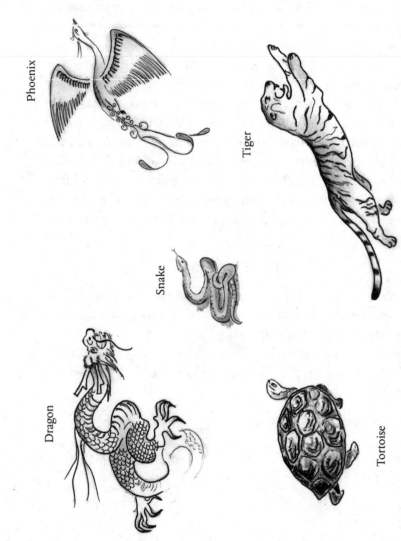

Phoenix

Tiger

Snake

Dragon

Tortoise

The Five Animals by Mariola McGrath

THE TORTOISE: SECURITY

The tortoise has a strong shell to protect it. It is placed at the rear, to give a sense of security. One tried to select a dwelling with a hill at the rear, making it safer from attack. In terms of modern homes, they should feel protected at the rear, perhaps by a high wall. If there was a wide open space at the back of our home, we would feel constantly on edge. Similarly, if we are sitting in a room, it feels more secure to have our backs to the wall. It feels very insecure to have our backs to an open space, or to a door.

One should avoid having water at the rear of one's home, as this harms the tortoise. Water at the rear creates disturbances in the flow of qi, and can make one feel drained.

In the bedroom, the head of the bed should not back to the door, as this can feel very insecure. The foot of the bed should face the door, so that one can see people coming in to the room. The bed should be in a protected position, tucked securely in a corner.

If the tortoise is absent from our home, we will tend to be nervous and unsettled. Our sleep may be restless, and we may wake unrefreshed. An imbalanced tortoise may affect the kidneys. The kidneys give us our base energy, so a deficiency will leave us feeling both drained, and unable to relax properly. A kidney deficiency will leave us "running on empty". The tortoise is known for longevity, and we must look after it if we want to live a long and healthy life. Often the root of cancer is kidney deficiency, so those with cancer should ensure that they have a healthy tortoise in their home.

THE DRAGON: HEIGHT

The dragon rests on the clouds, and by having an overview helps to create a sense of security. It sits on our left hand side. To the left of our home should be something slightly higher, such as some woods, or a high tree in the garden. In the bedroom, we can place a chest or wardrobe to the left of the bed. The dragon is associated with the liver organ, which is associated with planning and making decisions. When the dragon is not well, we can feel stagnant and unable to move forward and make decisions.

THE TIGER: PROTECTION

The tiger crouches low down on the right. It is essential for survival, but must be carefully controlled. Without the tiger we are very vulnerable, as it gives us clear boundaries and protection. The tiger is associated with the lungs, which also give us protection. Without our tiger, our immune system may be weakened. For those with cancer, it is essential to protect one's immunity.

One can have something like a shed or a garage to the right of the house. In the bedroom one can have a small bedside table on the right of the bed.

THE PHOENIX: INSPIRATION AND OPENNESS

One should have a nice open view at the front of one's home. Ideally one should be able to see into the distance: looking down into a valley is perfect. It is fine to have a view of water at the front. However, if the front of one's house looks onto a busy road, or onto tall buildings, one feels hemmed in and enclosed. One's imagination and inspiration is subdued. One's vision of life becomes restricted, and one's optimism is dimmed. The phoenix is associated with the heart, and with the spirit. One must be careful to nourish this aspect.

One should have a nice open phoenix aspect at work, to inspire creativity and help give a positive outlook. In Hong Kong, office blocks with a healthy phoenix often command a premium, as people recognise that this will promote successful business.

The ideal situation has the mountains at the rear, looking out into the bay.

THE SNAKE: CENTRE

The snake lies at the centre, at the very heart of the home. In traditional cultures this would have been the kitchen, where everyone gathered to share food. This area is associated with the earth element, which represents integration. By sharing this space, the people in the home develop oneness with each other, and harmony is created. We can think of a nice large farmhouse kitchen, with a big table around which everyone gathers. The room should be painted yellow, the colour of earth. People are naturally drawn to this area to socialise. There should not be a television in this area, as it prevents people from interacting with each other. Creating such an area at the heart of the home promotes harmony in the family.

Having such an area for meals also strengthens the digestive system. By providing a harmonious atmosphere it allows the digestive system to work more effectively. By encouraging people to linger and talk after the meal, it also allows the digestive system to do its work.

Having a healthy snake allows the qi to gather in the home, and therefore enhances the qi of those living there. Without a snake, the qi will tend to dissipate, and one will feel tired.

THE POSITION OF THE HOME

This can have a profound impact on one's health. The home should be surrounded by the five animals. Protection at the rear, and an open view at the front, are especially important.

One should also consider the position of roads around the house. If a road is directed at one's house, such as if one is living outside a bend in the road, this can create a feeling of tension. If you imagine a speeding car going off the road, would it hit your house? If so, there are likely to be negative energy lines rushing into the house, disturbing the energy there.

One should not live on a busy road, as this feels unsettling. The constant noise of cars over-stimulates one's nervous system and leaves one feeling tired. This is particularly important if one's kidneys are weak. On the other hand, it is good to locate one's business on a main road, as a strong flow of energy is good for business.

At the other extreme, one should avoid "dead end" cul-de-sacs, as these can feel stagnant. The energy has nowhere to flow, and ends up getting trapped and causing disturbances. This is very important to address if one has stagnant qi.

INTERNAL ARRANGEMENTS

A room should be arranged according to its purpose. A bedroom should be peaceful and uncluttered, with pale, restful colours. If one is prone to overheating, one can use a cooling colour such as light green in the bedroom. The bed should not be caught in an "energy draught", as this will create a restless sleep. As energy draught is a place between two openings, either windows or doors. The qi flow will be strong in these areas, and they are not appropriate for areas of sleep or relaxation. One should not sleep under beams, or under overhanging cupboards, as these can cause the energy to stagnate, and create a sense of unease. The back of the bed should be against a wall, to provide security. The bed should preferably be made of wood, rather than metal, as wood has softer energy. One should not have plants in the bedroom, as they compete with humans for oxygen during the night. One should not sleep under overhanging lights, as these cause energy disturbance.

On the other hand, a room which is used for work should be arranged to encourage the energy to flow freely. One can use more vibrant colours, and have more windows and light.

In the living room, one should also sit in a protected position, avoiding energy draughts between windows and doors. One should sit with one's back to the wall, and avoid having one's back to the door. Naughty children are often made to sit facing the wall, which is the most uncomfortable position in the room. They have no phoenix aspect at the front, and no protective tortoise aspect at the rear.

Of course, the above information is only a brief snapshot of the art of Feng Shui. We have only space to mention a few ideas from this extremely complex and detailed area of knowledge, which takes many years to master. The influence of one's surroundings has a profound impact on one's health, and should be taken into consideration, particularly if patients are not responding well to treatment. In this case one should consult a properly trained Feng Shui practitioner.

CONCLUSION

The state of a person's qi is a crucial determinant of their health. There are many ways to increase qi, and each person must find the best way to nourish their own qi. What works for some will not work for others. It is important that one finds a sense of joy in the work, as this is part of the process of healing. Having said that, it is also important to be persistent. In this chapter we have only given a brief outline of some ways to cultivate qi, which is by no means exhaustive.

Human beings have found countless ways to nourish and move their qi, even though most of the time we are not consciously doing so. Children naturally find things to do which nourish them and give them joy, such as playing games, drawing, dancing and singing. *These are the things which move their qi, and this is one reason why children are so full of vitality.* As we get older we often lose this sense of playfulness, which is so important for our qi. "Let the little children come unto me...for only those such as these will enter the Kingdom of Heaven."[139]

In conclusion, we mention one report of a woman who survived cancer, undertaking various complementary therapies. She had advanced (Stage IV) ovarian cancer, with widespread metastases, for which the survival rate at five years is almost unheard of in the literature. In 1978 she received a hysterectomy, but refused chemotherapy, and was given three months to live. She was symptom free until 1991, when another mass was discovered in her lower abdomen. Again, she refused chemotherapy, and decided to embark on her own intensive programme of mind–body therapies. The authors conclude that:

> We are not aware of any published report on long-term, disease-free survival of a patient with stage IV ovarian cancer and recurrent disease not treated by aggressive chemotherapy after surgery. The patient we describe is now 27 years after first diagnosis and recurrences and remains clinically free of disease. Based on this report and the data in the literature, we recommend further scientific research to assess the efficacy of CAM modalities for patients with cancer.[140]

In short, there are as many ways to cultivate qi as there are human beings.

---

139   *Holy Bible*, Matthew 19:14.
140   Lev-ari *et al. Integrative Cancer Therapies* 2006 Dec;5(4):395–9.

RESOURCES

Qi Gong

I am unaware of any registers outside China which list practitioners of external Qi gong. The following registers list teachers of internal Qi Gong exercises, but I am unable to certify that these teachers are of a good standard. The best tip is to ask your acupuncturist/Chinese herbalist for a recommendation.

When selecting a class, take careful note of the personality of the teacher. The best teachers are usually modest, down to earth, and friendly. Avoid anyone who seems to have a big ego, or who likes to demonstrate his "special powers". If you get a chance, talk to the students, and ask them how long they have been coming. A class with many long-standing students is a good sign. It is best to discuss your health with the teacher, and see whether he is comfortable with it.

UK

I am unaware of any national Qi Gong registers in the UK.

USA

The National Qigong Association (NQA) has a website with teacher listings: www.nqa.org.

CANADA

The Qi Gong Association has a website with teacher listings: http://qi.org.

AUSTRALIA

The Qi Gong Association has a website with teacher listings: http://qi.org.

Feng Shui

Properly qualified practitioners of this art are few and far between in the West, and I am not aware of any proper registers of practitioners. One therefore has to rely on word of mouth alone. There are many people who advertise themselves as practitioners, but who appear to have had very little training. Many of the "practitioner courses" on offer comprise only a few days training. When making enquiries, always ask how many years the person trained: a proper practitioner will have trained for many years.

CONCLUSION

This book has shown that cancer occurs as the result of many factors. Its manifestation in any one person reflects a pattern unique to her, and Chinese medicine seeks to identify that pattern. The book has argued that cancer reflects an imbalance in the *whole* person. It is not enough simply to cut out or poison the cancer itself, we must address *all* of the factors which have contributed to its development. It is necessary to seek the whole person, and to help her move towards harmony, both within herself, and with the rest of creation.

Chinese medicine is built on the understanding that there is a fundamental unity underlying creation. There is a thread holding the web of life together, a pattern in which all things play their part. By using Chinese medicine, one is enabled to access this unity, which is known as Tao. One is enabled to play one's full part in life, to become as whole a person as possible. In becoming full persons, we achieve harmony within ourselves, and with the rest of creation. We can use the analogy of an orchestra: each of us has an instrument to play in the "cosmic orchestra". We are all called to play our own parts, in harmony with all around us.

Chinese medicine itself is also a unity, and no strand is complete by itself. Herbs and diet nourish and strengthen our physical bodies, and help us become one with the earth which gives us life. Acupuncture helps to alleviate physical and mental suffering, promoting the harmonious movement of qi within ourselves, and between each other. Qi is a bridge between the physical and material worlds, and when it flows freely body and soul are integrated.

Through the arts of Qi Gong and Feng Shui we cultivate our qi further, and learn to harmonise our lives with the wider environment. Finally, through contemplating the words of those who were advanced in the pursuit of Tao, we strive to unify our spirits with the whole of creation. In this pursuit of the One we transcend our narrow selves and become more fully human. If one manages to achieve this, thoughts of illness and death no longer have the power to destroy our lives. If we can maintain our harmony in the face of the tiger, we have found harmony indeed.

CONTACTING THE AUTHOR

Please contact me by e-mail on: henry_mcgrath@blueyonder. co.uk; or via my website: henrymcgrath.com

INDEX